THE END OF SENILITY

Also by Dr. Arthur S. Freese

THE MIRACLE OF VISION
TURNING GRIEF INTO GROWTH
ARTHRITIS
HYPNOSIS FOR YOU
YOUR KIDNEYS
MANAGING YOUR DOCTOR
LOW BACK PAIN
OCCULT MEDICINE
EXECUTIVE LIFE-STYLE
PAIN
ASPIRIN AND YOUR HEALTH
HEADACHES
CAREERS IN THE MEDICAL SCIENCES
THE JOINT PROBLEM

THE END OF SENILITY

by Dr. Arthur S. Freese

ARBOR HOUSE
New York

 PUBLISHED IN THE UNITED STATES BY ARBOR HOUSE PUBLISHING COMPANY AND IN CANADA BY CLARKE, IRWIN & COMPANY, INC.

LIBRARY OF CONGRESS CATALOGUE CARD NUMBER: 77-90662

ISBN: 0-87795-173-X

MANUFACTURED IN THE UNITED STATES OF AMERICA

Contents

Or, as Robert Browning's Rabbi Ben Ezra proclaims:

> **Grow old along with me!**
> **The best is yet to be,**
> **The last of life, for which the first was made;**

ACKNOWLEDGEMENTS

SO MANY have helped and contributed both time and expertise to this book that only a few can be named and these will simply be noted alphabetically, individuals first, and then the organizations and their special people. MY THANKS:

To Dr. Ewald W. Busse—Professor of Psychiatry at Duke University and Founding Director of its Center for the Study of Aging and Human Development—whose wisdom, compassion, and vast knowledge of psychiatry and the elderly have been so generously shared both here and in numerous other endeavors in the past.

To Dr. Robert N. Butler—Director of the National Institute on Aging—whose interest in geropsychiatry led him to pioneer and provide a much needed public voice for the elderly and who gave so freely of his time and thinking.

To Dr. James C. Folsom—Director of ICD Rehabilitation and Research Center and former head of Rehabilitation Medicine for the entire Veterans Administration—who shared with me his development of the exciting turn-around new treatment, Reality Orientation, that has proved so important in the fight against "senility."

To Dr. Leslie S. Libow—Medical Director of the Jewish Institute for Geriatric Care of New Hyde Park, N.Y.—for giving his time and expertise as one of the leading and very few geriatricians of whom the United States can boast.

To Dr. F. Marott Sinex—Co-Director of the Boston University Gerontology Center and Professor of Biochemistry—for his expertise, honesty, and generosity with time taken from a very busy schedule.

And for those whose names must be linked with their organizations even though they deserve separate mention—again in alphabetical order: MY THANKS:

To Gilbert F. Martin, Manager of Magazine Relations, and his American Medical Association for untiring cooperation and help over many years.

To Robert L. Robinson, Director of Public Affairs, and his American Psychiatric Association, for generosity in supplying help and materials both here and in many other endeavors.

To Mona Marie Olean, Public Information Officer, and her American Psychological Association, in appreciation of so much cooperation here as in many other works.

To Joe Sigler, Public Relations Director, and his Duke University Center for the Study of Aging and Human Development, with thanks for their generous and very considerable help.

To Daniel S. Rogers, Information Officer, for his frequent help and that of his two organizations—the NIA Gerontology Research Center in Baltimore and the Gerontólogical Society.

To Jane E. Shure, Public Information Officer, and her National Institute on Aging, for their cooperation and generous supply of information whenever needed.

Introduction: The Glittering New Hope

Here is truly good news: the story of the magnificent triumph of modern medical science over some of man's most feared and ancient enemies. King Lear shuddered at the approach of old age and cried out in anguish: "O! Let me not be mad, not mad, sweet heaven"—and for the first time since man appeared on this planet the terrifying shadow of the madness that man has learned to call "senility" has been lifted. At long last we can truly speak of the end of senility, and of the obsolescence, as well, of "old age" as we have always known it. Man naturally ages and does become aged, but he need no longer become "an old man" with all the traditional connotations of incapacity and sadly diminished usefulness, even uselessness, that attach to it. There has been a turnabout in man's life span—but even more important he now has the opportunity to add life to his years rather than merely empty years to his life.

That is why this book has been written—to make available to modern knowledge of how to increase *both* life and years, to offer facts, preventions and cures, to lift the depressing and frightening shadow of past myths. It is a book for *everyone*, for while all of us would like to live long, none of us wants to become "old" or "senile"—and it is now actually possible both to prevent and cure what has been known as "senility," to convert old age into late middle age, to strengthen and improve memory, to help both men and women enjoy a rich and potent sexual life all of their lives, to hold out an exciting promise for the future.

Not even our most enthusiastic and optimistic medical scientists claim that we will become a nation of Methuselahs, but the "graying of America" is already much evident. One in every ten Americans is already past the age of sixty-five, and those over the age of seventy-five constitute the fastest-growing segment of America's population. The balance continues to swing in favor of the over-sixty-fives and will do so well into the twenty-first century—and no one can really be faulted for thinking of Methuselah when the 1970 census showed more than one hundred thousand Americans reported being over the age of one hundred!

Nevertheless, there is a strong problem of ageism in our society—a form of prejudice against the elderly that is just as terrible and damaging as any racism or sexism. It is an insidious condition, based largely on falsehoods, but so prevalent that its victims themselves tend to believe in it—and convert the falsehoods into self-fulfilling prophecies. By understanding the reality and the effects of these prejudices, it is possible for those who have passed the mythical cutoff age of sixty-five to deal with their own reactions to this pressure—and to fight back against the myths with information and facts instead of submitting docilely.

Old age is obsolete today; in the face of current reality,

the concept has become outmoded. In fact, the French have a much better expression for it—"The Third Age," following "The First Age" of schooling and "The Second Age" of intense activity. "The Third Age" is a particular developmental period, a creative and often highly productive time of life, a period filled with rich rewards. We will explore many of them here—the true potentialities for those over sixty-five, what they (man or woman) can really do, how they can deal with the myths and illusions that have so long made them behave like "old people" simply because society said they should.

The good life demands good health, however—and the older person must also learn not only how to make the most of what is essentially vigorous health, but how to find proper medical care. This can be a problem: most physicians are neither knowledgeable about nor comfortable with older patients, and the result literally can be the difference between life and death. Older and younger patients can react in sharply different ways to drugs, for instance, or to diseases such as appendicitis and heart attacks, and all too often doctors are insufficiently trained to recognize the difference. The consequences can be tragic, not only because of possible death, but because the symptoms sometimes mimic those that we associate with "senility," and so the patient ends up misdiagnosed as "hopeless," condemned to the half-life of a mental institution or nursing home—when all he needs is simple, good medical care. In the chapters to come, we'll explore how and where to find the best medical care—and the best way to utilize it when it's found.

We'll also look at where to get help for sexual problems and see what happens to sexuality after sixty-five—how, in fact, it can become richer and more satisfying with age, a matter of growth and development despite the cruel, bigoted, and invariably mistaken "jokes." We'll also look at the emotional problems of the older person; how to cope with retirement; the dangers of drugs for older citizens; the warning signals of certain major mental problems that can be reversed if caught in time; and how to combat that most common American mental health problem, depression. There's even an exciting new approach that promises help for those who are actually afflicted with dementia. For this is a book of promise and hope, a book that says you can grow older but never "old," that having *more* years does not mean having *less* life.

Or, as Robert Browning's Rabbi Ben Ezra proclaims:

Grow old along with me!
The best is yet to be,
The last of life for which the first was made.

CHAPTER 1

Why Old Age is Now Obsolete

BENJAMIN FRANKLIN was in his seventies when he helped write the Declaration of Independence and our Constitution, negotiated with France for military aid, and concluded our peace treaty with Great Britain—and eighty-three when he invented bifocal eyeglasses. U.S. Supreme Court Justice Oliver Wendell Holmes was in his eighties when he wrote some of his classic legal opinions, and only resigned from the Court when he was ninety-one. Leopold Stokowski was still conducting orchestral performances at the age of ninety-five. Picasso and Casals were both active into their nineties. Michelangelo began his "Pieta" when he was seventy-five and the designing of St. Peter's cupola when he was eighty-three . . . we could go on and on.

And it is not only the rare geniuses who can achieve this sort of longevity. Dr. Roy M. Hamlin, a Danville, Illinois, psychologist on the staff of the Veterans Administration Hospital, makes a brilliant and impressive plea for an entirely new definition of old age ("old age in flux," he calls it) and proves his point with everyday cases: an eighty-one-year-old woman who cares for her own house and rides a power mower to cut about five acres of grass. Forty retired men and women ranging in age from sixty to eighty-four in Grenoble, France, bicycle thirty miles regularly through the adjacent French High Alps of southeastern France where their university city is located. My own grandmother was ninety-two when my grandfather died and she gave up her home to come and live with us; hearing radio programs regularly for the first time, she became annoyed that she didn't speak English better and began working at it—her English was still improving when she died several years later. And a friend's uncle was still making trips abroad to see the world until his death at the age of ninety-seven.

And so it goes—with such examples and patterns before us we must begin to rethink our conventional American beliefs and concepts about "old age" and even about aging itself. To do this, we should first take a look at how these beliefs evolved.

Man has always been frightened of old age, with its specter of disabilities and losses and its eventual outcome, death. To protect himself from such fears ancient man struck back in the only way at his command—with myths and fables, promises and recorded hopes. The Bible tells of Methuselah who lived 969 years, and records the offer of long life as the ultimate reward for obedience to its religion and its God. Greek mythology reveals the antiquity of mankind's dream of immortality and its fears of aging with the legend of Eos and Tithonus. Eos, the goddess of the dawn, fell in love with Tithonus, a handsome but mortal youth, and carried him off to become her lover and the father of her two children. So enamored was she that she begged Zeus to make Tithonus immortal, but being somewhat scatterbrained she forgot to ask for eternal youth as well. Thus, with time, Tithonus aged and turned gray, and Eos soon lost interest in him. He became enfeebled and began to babble endlessly and Eos locked him in a room to be quit of him—the perfect picture of old age as Shakespeare represented it in *As You Like It*: "second childishness, and mere oblivion / Sans teeth, sans eyes, sans taste, sans everything." These unhappy pictures have hung on.

The aged in society have been treated in as many different ways as there are cultures. They have been fed to flesh-eating dogs and worshipped as gods, thrown off a cliff and rendered absolute obedience. The ancient Hebrews believed that it was only evildoers that died young, the Greeks believed that those who died at a young age were the beloved of their gods. Eastern peoples venerated their elders—the title "Sheikh" (accorded leaders and chiefs) actually comes from the Arabic *shaikh* meaning "old man"—and the Senate, the highest governing body in western societies, gets its name from the Latin *senex*, meaning "old" or "old man." Yet in the United States the "old man" is looked at askance.

Dr. Robert N. Butler, geropsychiatrist and Director of the National Institute on Aging (NIA), sums up our problem this way: "Americans suffer from a personal and institutionalized prejudice against older people. Although this may be a primitive, universal dread of aging true in all cultures, it is reinforced and thus more striking in our own." And Dr. John H. Budd, 1977-1978 President of the American Medical Association (AMA), outlines the overall problem: "Old people suffer from a contagious disease that is found in no medical dictionary. It is attitude. Lying outside the medical dictionary, this contagion cannot be cured by medicine alone. All the forces of society must help relieve it—and society means each of us in each of our daily roles."

Since every one of us is involved—either as older people or as people who are becoming older each day—let us examine the realities: how long man lives today, what "old age" is and what goes on in the process of aging, what ageism and the myths of aging are, how and why we are prejudiced against the elderly. And, last of all—why aging is now obsolete.

HOW LONG DOES MAN LIVE AND WHAT IS "OLD AGE"?

Man's life span on this planet has changed markedly since his earliest days. The average Neanderthal seems to have lived only some twenty years; in classical Greece and Rome, men scraped together a little more time, making the average life span twenty-seven or twenty-eight; the medieval Englishman managed thirty-two; at the turn of our own century the average age was roughly forty-seven—and then it began to rise sharply. Although it hit a plateau about 1954, it is now about seventy-one years.

More significant perhaps to the actual meaning of "old age" is the fact that four out of five Neanderthals were dead by the age of thirty; and all were gone by fifty. Our own first national census in 1790 found half of all Americans to be sixteen years or younger and less than one in five Americans reaching the biblical three score years and ten—while today half of our citizens are twenty-nine or less and more than four out of five can anticipate living longer than seventy.

Today it is the centenarian—the one hundred-year-old person—who draws startled gasps. People are fascinated by reports of 4,500 to 5,000 centenarians in the Soviet Republic of Georgia in the Caucasus and numerous centenarians in the small independent state of Hunza set amidst the towering peaks of the Pakistani-Chinese border. Most Americans tend to forget, however, that for all the charm of distance and strangeness, more than 106,000 *Americans* (as Dr. Butler points out) reported themselves as being over one hundred years old in the 1970 census.

In addition, skeptical voices have been raised about some of these reports. A distinguished Russian gerontologist, Dr. Zhores A. Medvedev, questions the Russian ages, calling attention to the absence of birth records, the rapid rise in the numbers of these self-declared centenarians, the greater proportion of male centenarians as compared to female (the opposite of what one would expect), and the marked discrepancy between the claimed age and the proven life expectancy of others in their own society. There has even been some proven falsification as well.

Dr. George H. Gallup, father of scientific public opinion polling, also warns of being deceived by many of these stories, since he has found absolute correlation between illiteracy and claims of length of life: "We figure that when they got to be eighty they started counting the years by tens—and in this country the same thing happens." As Dr. Gallup warns: "Unless you have birth certificates or positive proof don't believe it when someone says he's 100 or 126 or 146 or whatever!" In 1973, Moscow announced the death of Shirali Mislimov, a Caucasian peasant of 168 years, believed to have been the world's oldest man (his 105-year-old wife survived him)—but the Soviets also admitted that Mislimov had no birth records. The 1977 edition of the *Guinness Book of World Records* finds that the oldest *authenticated* age was that of a woman born at Stark, New York, on May 8, 1815, who lived more than 113 years to her death on December 4, 1928.

In any case, our age mix has been changing drastically in the United States. In 1900, three million Americans—4 percent of the population—were over the age of sixty-five; today the figure is twenty-three million, more than 10 percent—and of that number more than ten million are over the age of seventy-three and one million are eighty-five or older. In fact, the age group over seventy-five years old is the fastest-growing segment of our entire population.

What then is the "normal" human life span? Dr. Butler sees it as perhaps "somewhere between 100 and 120 years"—and most gerontologists (those engaged in the scientific study of aging) are inclined to agree. And "old age"—well, who knows? The answer has been as variable as our societies, the ultimate test usually being man's ability to function physically and mentally. It used to be thirty or forty years. Ancient Chinese scholars, though a little vague, wrote of the sixties and the age of seventy as fulfilling the concept, while Pythagoras set it as sixty.

President Franklin Roosevelt selected an intermediate year, sixty-five, as the time for Social Security benefits and retirement, and so, presumably, as "old age" (in actuality, the age of sixty-five was chosen long before FDR. In 1889, Germany's Chancellor Otto von Bismarck put the "Old Age and Survivors Pension Act" through the Reichstag with an arbitrary cutoff figure of sixty-five—even though Bismarck himself was then a brilliant and physically active seventy-four!). And for some time the young have even been setting their own concept of old age with their loudly proclaimed, "Don't trust anyone over thirty!"

Whatever the specific age, the cultural effect of choosing a figure for purely legislative purposes, with no scientific or medical reasons, has been that Americans today "feel old" at a certain age because society officially says they are. As we shall see later, this societal attitude is a highly powerful force in its members' thinking. It will be interesting to see what the effect will be of the 1977 Congressional ban on mandatory retirement for most workers before the age of seventy, and how long it will need to take hold.

WHAT IS AGING?

There are different kinds of "aging." The biologist is interested in how the cells and tissues of the organism run down with the passage of time; the physician looks for increased susceptibility to disease or special disorders as the person moves from infancy through the life cycle; the sociologist thinks in terms of the society's influence on a person in a particular age group; the psychologist looks at emotional changes and at such special faculties as memory. The criteria can vary enormously.

So can the measurements. Aging is at best an uneven

process—one of my sixty-year-old patients had the heart of a woman twenty years younger but the skin of a woman of eighty—and inconsistencies in development can be found in most people to a greater or lesser degree. It's rare that any of us are like the wonderful one-horse shay, made of such perfectly matched materials that it ran for a hundred years and a day and then every part collapsed simultaneously.

Perhaps the most bizarre example of inconsistent aging is a medical condition called "progeria," a fortunately rare but exceedingly tragic disorder. As of this writing, there are fewer than sixty recorded cases of this disease, in which infants become old virtually before their parents' eyes: they develop thinning gray hair and baldness; dried-out, wrinkled skin; fragile bone structure and even the heart diseases of the elderly; finally dying in their teens. Not long ago, a well-known medical magazine showed a series of pictures of an infant boy at six months of age and then at a year and a half; he seemed normal—but his picture at eight years old was that of a balding, aging man in his late sixties. He died of congestive heart failure long before he even reached his teens, the image of a sagging, wrinkled man in his seventies or eighties.

Another rare condition—Werner's syndrome—appears in the late teens and also involves rapid and very premature aging until the victim dies at about the age of forty from what is seeming old age. There have been only some 130 cases of this tragic syndrome recorded.

Except in science fiction no one has really entertained any hope of changing chronological aging, but throughout our history man has recurrently fantasized about somehow delaying the onset of old age—usually in the context of sexual vigor. The Old Testament's King David obviously believed—and tried—the Oriental concept that rejuvenation was possible by absorbing youthful vigor from young women, as did the Romans. The medieval Europeans had other ideas, though; they sought the fountain of youth. In fact, Ponce de Leon was able to finance and mount an entire expedition to the New World just for that purpose in 1512. He discovered Florida instead. (Maybe he was not so far off after all. Many older Americans go to Florida to seek renewal of their youth. In fact, there is a group of men between the ages of seventy and ninety in St. Petersburg who gather regularly to play baseball—and perhaps succeed where Ponce de Leon failed.)

Biologists generally define aging as the steady and increasing loss of the capacity to function that living tissues undergo with the passage of time, though there is disagreement as to whether these changes should be dated from the maturation of the organism or from shortly after conception. This process, in turn, has been broken down by many scientists into two categories—primary and secondary aging. Primary aging consists of the biological processes built into our genes—the inborn deleterious changes resulting from the passage of time alone. This kind may not be recognizable in everyone nor does it proceed at any uniform or standard rate. Secondary aging, on the other hand, is a matter of those biological processes and disabilities that result from injuries, diseases, stress, and environmental influences. As such, they are, of couse, highly unpredictable.

Frankly, we just don't know what really *causes* aging or what these biological processes are. There are intriguing theories. One is that as a clock runs down, so do we—we have only so much energy and that's it. Another simple theory is that noxious or detrimental products accumulate in our cells during life until they eventually become damaging or overwhelming.

Dr. F. Marott Sinex, Co-Director of Boston University's Gerontology Center and professor of biochemistry, regards aging as something that is biologically programmed with a very real biochemical limitation to the length of our lives. Another and rather recent theory is that as cells grow old they develop errors in reproducing or copying themselves and so lose both functional efficiency and the ability to repair themselves as efficiently as before. This process continues until the breakdown and failure of the total organism finally results "with age."

Dr. Denham Harman, University of Nebraska professor of medicine, is the founder of the free radical theory. "Free radicals" are highly unstable atoms, bits of molecules missing an electron—which function as very reactive chemical agents. They will seize on any cells available—and can alter them permanently. Dr. Harman believes that: "Free radical reactions shorten life span, contribute to the development of cancer (at least some forms), dampen immune responses, and most likely play a significant role in the degradation of the central nervous [brain and spinal cord] and cardiovascular [heart and blood vessel] systems." But like so much else in biology and medicine today, this theory is not fully accepted by any means.

Another possibility is that longevity may simply be the reward for having inherited a superior immune system. The body's immune system is the complex bodily defense mechanism that protects against infection by attacking foreign elements (bacteria or viruses or whatever) that invade the body. This system weakens with time, however, so that the older person has a lowered resistance to infection. In addition, the passage of time presents an increasing likelihood of autoimmune reactions, in which the immune system turns upon its owner and actually attacks the body's organs or tissues (this is a possible cause of arthritis and of certain very serious brain diseases or dementias, for example).

Stress and traumatic life experiences too, may shorten life. The outstanding world authority on stress, Dr. Hans Selye, Director of Montreal University's Institute of Experimental Medicine and Surgery, believes that human beings have just so much "adaptation energy" that we can use to cope with the trauma and stresses of life. When this is finally all burned up by too much stress, whether psychological or physical, the final stress leads to death.

But society itself takes a toll too in the form of . . .

AGEISM AND THE MYTHS OF AGING

They're "crocks . . . boobies . . . crones . . . old fogies." They're "over the hill" and "out to pasture." That's how America regards its citizens over sixty-five. As Dr. Eric Pfeiffer, Duke University professor of psychiatry, points out, aging "has been given a bad press . . . presented as one hopeless, unremitting downward drift into despair, deprivation, and desolation." This is what NIA Director Butler terms "ageism"—the stereotypes and prejudices held by our society about the aged, arising from our natural human fear of physical and mental decline and death and from our society's strong youth orientation. Out of this prejudice have come most of the myths that plague the elderly and confuse society.

The elderly are viewed as weak, incompetent, unproductive, uncreative; they can't change or learn new things; they're rigid and intellectually sterile. As we've seen over and over again, however, older people today are creative, active and prolific. As a contributing editor to *Modern Maturity* magazine, I have interviewed dozens of the major figures of our century, all over the age of sixty-five and most of them in their seventies and eighties—Lowell Thomas, Dr. Milton Eisenhower, Dr. George Gallup, Faith Baldwin, the Reverend Norman Vincent Peale, Nobelist Dr. Albert Szent-Gyorgyi, historian Bruce Catton, poet Mark Van Doren; dancers and religious leaders, novelists and cartoonists, men and women, scientists and architects and psychiatrists. One thing stands out: all were alert, active, creative, and productive, and clearly all would be (or were) until the very end.

In point of fact, this concept that the over-sixty-five person is incapable of useful work is relatively new—in 1900 an estimated 70 percent of American men over sixty-five were working. Although by now this is down to around 20 percent, still, as recently as 1971, the Bureau of Labor found that 1,780,000 people over sixty-five were working full time and another 1,257,000 part time.

HOW AGING HAS BECOME OBSOLETE

In 1955, twenty-one National Institute of Mental Health (NIMH) investigators representing a broad range of medical sciences began an eleven-year study of human aging, using healthy men living in their communities (not in institutions) ranging in age from sixty-five to ninety-one, with a mean age of seventy-one (as many were above this age as below). The investigators found them "generally flexible [with] alert, keen minds . . . constructive, resourceful, and optimistic," and the internists doing the physical examinations were very impressed by their excellent health and vigor.

A larger, much more comprehensive study was also begun in 1955 by the Duke University Center for the Study of Aging and Human Development, using nearly 300 men and women in a broad ethnic and socioeconomic mix between the ages of sixty and ninety (500 more people were added to the study in 1968). The results? Dr. George L. Maddox, Director of the Duke Center, sums them up:

"There is substantial potential for effective living well into the individual seventies. Our psychological testing has revealed a quite remarkable stability in a healthy older person's capacity to respond to an I.Q. test or to learn new things . . . the origins of the saying 'old dogs can't learn' lies more in the lack of motivation to learn than in the ability. Our society simply doesn't provide learning opportunities for older individuals, nor does it encourage them to continue learning."

This American concept of aging must be changed. As we have seen, the men or women today who are sixty to eighty-five, even ninety, are on the same plateau as those in their fifties years ago. Instead of "old age," we should recognize it as late *middle* age. Even with such developments of our time as atomic energy and the conquest of space, still, as Dr. Roy M. Hamlin points out, "the two most important developments are these: longer life and increasing competence in old age."

He also points out how in the past century the average life span has increased more than in the preceding two thousand years, and anyone equating chronic illness with the aged makes virtually the same error as equating juvenile delinquency with adolescence. "The chronological age that marks the average beginning of old age has been moved ahead, perhaps from sixty-five to eighty-five . . . Never before has there been 'an entire new race' as we have today." In short, old age is becoming, in a very real sense, obsolete—and life may be good, useful and rewarding until the very end.

But to make old age obsolete it is also essential to wipe out another of the terribly destructive myths of this period—and that is the subject of our next chapter.

CHAPTER 2

Putting an End to Senility—The Myths, The Errors and The Facts

J WAS an executive in a large East Coast city when he found even routine daily tasks too much for him. He seemed to slow down both physically and mentally and increasingly withdrew inside himself, shutting out people and events in the world about him. He slept little and at times seemed confused and disoriented, unsure of what day or date it was, sometimes forgetting even the names of those about him. He began to drift about his own home, aimlessly and distractedly; his dress and appearance turned slovenly; he even neglected bodily care.

R was a housewife in a small midwestern community when she showed up in the chief local department store unkempt and obviously confused, ignorant of where she was although she'd shopped in that store virtually all her life. Unable to recall why or how she'd gotten there, even uncertain of her own name and address, she wandered about in aimless circles until she finally broke out in tears of despair. Recognized by the store personnel, she was finally sent home with a friend.

In both instances, the family doctor was consulted, but medical diagnoses are all too often determined not by the real medical or psychiatric condition but by the age of the sufferer and the doctor's own prejudices and lack of expertise—his ageism. As a result, the diagnosis of such a condition (both J and R suffered from the same disorder) can offer the victim and the family either a hopeful outlook with the promise of amelioration—or one that virtually condemns the victim to a hopeless, steadily deteriorating life in an institution.

If J and R are in their forties, for instance, the doctor usually makes a quick, correct diagnosis of depression—which seriously affects as many as 15 percent of all American adults—and then promptly takes active steps to utilize all of modern psychiatry's weapons against this disorder. If these unfortunates should be in their sixties or seventies or older, however, they are most likely to be regarded as hopeless, given no active treatment and condemned to a lifetime of institutionalization in a nursing home or mental hospital as "senile."

This is because the medical profession in the United States has, for the most part, little training, expertise, or interest in geriatrics, the medical specialty concerned with the problems and the care of those in their sixties and beyond, despite the fact that this rapidly growing segment of our population comprises roughly one out of every nine Americans. It is so important that older persons obtain adequate, competent medical care that Chapter 7 is devoted entirely to ways in which people can identify the right physicians, together with the ways to find them.

Misdiagnoses of the over-sixty-five person can be caused by medical problems as well as psychiatric problems such as depression. Take the seventy-five-year-old woman whose heart no longer pumps as efficiently as it should. With reduced blood and nourishment going to her brain, she may be a little fuzzy and forget some meals, causing anemia and still less oxygen to the brain. A hot day and dehydration—and the woman is found wandering in the streets, confused and disoriented, unable to recall where she is or even her home address.

If that woman's daughter fails to get a really competent doctor he may (as so many do) automatically say "Oh—she's getting senile" and dash off a prescription for tranquilizers while telling the family that nothing more can be done—even advising institutionalization. With this, the woman can only drift steadily downhill until irreversible damage is done to her brain and recovery is impossible. A knowledgeable physician, however, will carefully examine the woman, diagnose her heart condition (mild congestive heart failure) and treat it with the many effective drugs available. The woman will quickly respond, the "senility" will disappear, and she will be back to functioning normally for the foreseeable future.

Or take the case of A, in his late seventies, who suddenly became confused and markedly disoriented. The doctor said "senile" and advised a nursing home. He never discovered that A had had a mild heart attack because the doctor wasn't aware that the older person often doesn't have the classic symptoms of chest, arm, or neck pains, or even shortness of breath. As a result, a common, treatable medical disorder was allowed to become a destructive and irreversible mental condition.

Vast numbers of cases of what doctors and public alike so loosely term "senility" are actually matters of missed and neglected medical conditions ranging from mild heart conditions to depression, anemia to appendicitis, malnutrition to thyroid conditions, improperly prescribed medication, to viral infections. Both an older person's symptoms for a wide variety of diseases, and many of his reactions, can be markedly different from the textbook cases of a young adult—just as the fever that will make an adolescent or young adult merely uncomfortable can throw an infant into convulsions.

Before we go into the matter of senility, however, let's look at the organ from which this entire problem springs.

YOUR MAGNIFICENT BRAIN

It all began some 3.4 billion years ago with the appearance of the earliest known form of life on earth. Evidence of this life has only recently been uncovered in South Africa: some 200 cells, so small they had to be enlarged 1600 times—400 of them put in a line would only be the thickness of a dime. And in the heart of Ethiopia an international team of anthropologists, headed by a professor from Cleveland's Case Western Reserve University, has found upper and lower fossil jaws that seem to date the beginnings of man himself back almost five million years.

It has taken all this time to develop man's unbelievable

brain, a relatively small organ not much bigger than your clenched fist that still puzzles and awes our scientists. A little more than a century ago, a Cornell University biology professor, Burt Green Wilder, started a brain collection because it was then believed that one's mental capacities—intelligence, talents, training—could be recognized simply by examining the outer surface of the brain, what is often called the gray matter or the cerebral cortex. Cornell scientists accumulated their brains from a wide variety of men and women and busied themselves measuring and weighing, probing the depth and the length of that organ's convolutions to detect which areas controlled particular talents or abilities.

When Wilder retired in 1910, the Cornell Brain Association had 430 brains, including those of an alcoholic and "an erotic German," a physician and a murderer, a poet and a thief, a "bright schoolboy," and "an idiot"—even that of Helen Hamilton Gardener, a prominent women's suffrage leader. Born in 1833, Ms. Gardener was angered by a neurologist's statement that a woman's brain was inferior and struggled to disprove it by willing her brain to Cornell. While it was large, it was not as large as that of a compulsive murderer (believer to be the second largest on record). As with other outmoded concepts, this interest, too, faded away nearly a half-century ago.

Nor was it too long ago that scientists still thought that unraveling the brain's secrets would only be a matter of tediously and miscroscopically tracing out the nerve cells—the neurons—as one does a somewhat complex telephone system with its intricate connections and massive switchboards. This simplistic interpretation has given way to the current recognition that the brain is much more like a computerized ultrasophisticated radio-TV system of such complexity that our most advanced electronic engineer could not envisage it in his wildest dreams. Despite our electron microscopes with their more-than-a-million-times magnification, and the radioisotopes that broadcast their information as they pass through the intricate and delicate network of blood vessels that permeate the brain, and our advanced biochemical techniques and knowhow—we still have only just begun to glimpse something of the brain's fantastic complexities.

The entire human body consists of an estimated sixty trillion cells—but the brain alone boasts some twelve billion neurons (nerve cells) and an additional one hundred billion so-called "glia cells" whose function is still unclear—and atop it all lies that supreme achievement of nature, the human cerebral cortex. Comprising about half the weight of the entire nervous system, the cortex is a wrinkled cover, about one-tenth of an inch thick, of soft gray tissue that, if stretched out, would be some three feet long and two feet wide. The cortex is densely packed with neurons and glia cells, and the figures are mind-boggling: the entire brain is only three pounds of deeply convoluted shiny jelly, but a cubic inch contains one hundred million cells and a column the thickness of a pencil holds some 50,000 neurons.

It's in these individual neurons and their connections that the secrets of the brain diseases—the senile dementias so feared by man—are thought to lie, so let's look a little closer at them. Neurons are strangely chubby cells that adopt a wide variety of shapes and sizes, ranging up to several feet in length, although still less than 1/100 of an inch in diameter—and they haven't actually changed very much in the last half-billion years. In both shape and function, human neurons are nearly identical to those of the lizard, for example.

The cell body of the neuron is virtually a miniaturized chemical manufacturing system, so active that it needs an estimated fifteen billion atoms of oxygen a second. Stop its oxygen supply for ten seconds and the neuron is so affected you lose consciousness. This, of course, is the reason why any interference with the brain's blood supply—a heart condition or anemia or arteriosclerosis—produces so severe an effect on consciousness, causing confusion and disorientation.

Messages (neural impulses, essentially tiny bursts of electricity) come into the neuron through filamentous extensions, usually-short, called dendrites and are conducted on to the next neuron through a single long filament coming out of the cell body called an axon. There is no actual physical contact between neurons, however. The axon ends in a tiny knob at a gap called a synapse; less than one-millionth of an inch of space separates the axon of one neuron from the dendrites of the next. When the impulse is brought by the dendrite to the cell body it goes out along the axon to its synaptic knob where the impulse somehow releases chemicals—neurotransmitters—that travel across the synapse to open pores in the cell membrane of the adjoining neuron and there start another neural impulse off on its way.

These synapses are one-way switches that act to control the flood of impulses (sensations and information of all kinds from skin and organs and tissues) that pour into the central nervous system—tens of thousands of impulses reach the brain every second. By letting through only the important and meaningful signals, the synapses act as the policemen of the central nervous system and keep the enormous traffic under control to prevent the brain from being overwhelmed and throwing the person into an epileptic convulsion. So important are these synapses that there are some 500 trillion of them in the brain; some neurons possess almost a quarter of a million synapses each.

WHAT HAPPENS TO THE BRAIN WITH AGING

Information about the brain is limited by the fact that doctors can't do a biopsy—cut out a chunk of tissue—for study as they do with the skin or muscle or other tissues and organs that are readily accessible and can replace their lost cells. Neurons are irreplaceable and this fact is probably the basis of the physical, "organic" changes or damage in the brain. Once we have grown our full complement (by about the age of ten), that's it—we can never replace damaged neurons or grow new ones as we do with our skin as its cells wear off or age and die.

The result is that pathologists can only really study the brain after its owner has died and so much is still mysterious—but even so, a variety of things are known. For example, you've probably read the widely published statement that 100,000 neurons die each day. The experts statement that 100,000 neurons die each day. The experts ridicule such a figure. As Dr. Sinex says: "That's just some science writer who recalculated some old data." In actual fact, the loss of neurons depends on the part of the brain and whose estimates we want to use. For example, Dr.

Robert D. Terry, chairman of pathology at Albert Einstein College of Medicine and a leading authority on the brain and its diseases, calls attention to the figures he feels are correct: these show a 40 to 50 percent cell loss following one hundred years of normal aging, depending on the area of the brain—some parts don't seem to show any loss at all, ever.

Other changes, too, seem to occur and it's commonly felt that there is some shrinkage of the brain with age: a 5 percent weight loss by the time the person reaches seventy, which may increase to 20 percent by the nineties—but this is not invariable. Just what such observations mean is debatable, however—no one really knows, for example, if loss of neurons actually causes the slower reaction times prevalent in many older people. Certainly it's easy to point to many people in their eighties and nineties who show no change in intellectual capacity. As there is evidently a vast oversupply of neurons to protect against loss (since they are irreplaceable) such loss may not be significant anyway. In fact, the highly intelligent person seems to show considerably less difference and decline in overall ability with age than those with lesser intellectual capacities.

So what exactly is "senility" and where does it come from?

SENILITY: ITS REALITY AND MYTHOLOGY

As mentioned, the word senility has the same origin as the word "Senate"—the Latin *senex* meaning "old" or "old man." It first appeared in the English language in 1791—according to the *Oxford English Dictionary*—

when Boswell in his *Johnson* wrote of a person's consciousness of senility, and since then it has attained a certain respectability as a result of its nearly two centuries of usage by public and medical profession alike. The term carries a seeming scientific air—and patients listen with respect when the physician weightily pronounces a person "senile." So impressive and fearsome is such a "diagnosis" that patients and their loved ones are unfortunately overawed and hesitate to insist on a more specific and genuinely scientific medical diagnosis.

In actual cold medical and scientific fact there is no such thing as "senility"! Dr. Sinex says, "I never use the word," while Dr. Leslie S. Libow, Medical Director of Long Island's Jewish Institute for Geriatric Care, points out that, "It does not exist in the medical literature," and Dr. Butler, who has long and openly fought against the myth of senility, says of the term: "It has no real medical legitimacy and it's not used in any diagnostic nomenclature—but none the less it is used in an everyday manner by doctors and public alike and covers the waterfront—which is regrettable."

There is no such disease as "senility"—but there are more than a hundred possible different conditions whose causes lead to symptoms that we mistakenly, tragically picture as "senility." The picture is one of mental confusion and disorientation (as to time or place or both), dizziness and lack of self-care, forgetfulness, impairment of intellectual functioning and judgement, and inability to carry out even such everyday tasks as paying bills or going to the store. Even worse, this "diagnosis" carries with it implications of irreversibility, futility and hopelessness; and, overriding it all, the belief held so commonly and mistakenly by public and physicians alike that senility is the inevitable price of age, of daring to live beyond the age of sixty-five or the biblical three score and ten.

Among the worst aspects of this diagnosis is the fact that it is used today as a form of verbal shorthand to hide the ugly face of prejudice—of ageism—and to permit many physicians to avoid the need to diagnose and treat the over-sixty-five patient with the same care, thoroughness, and consideration that is accorded the adolescent, the young adult, or even the "middle-aged" patient. Dr. Butler has found it to be a particularly convenient term for physicians who don't want to spare the time for older women patients.

Dr. Butler—like so many other gerontologists, geriatricians, and geropsychiatrists—would like to see the end of "senility," this pseudoscientific term used as a catchall for disorders virtually none of which have anything specific to do with aging: "If I had my way, we would not even use the word 'senility,' but it is so deeply ingrained in the language that it's probably a fool's paradise to imagine getting rid of it—if we have proper education of our medical students regarding human aging this will go a long way toward clearing up the confusion in the minds of both the public and the doctors with regard to so-called 'senility'."

"Senility" is in fact simply a farce—a myth, a superstition—that has no place in either modern scientific medicine or in the thinking of today's America. The public's insistence upon an adequate specific diagnosis—congestive heart failure or anemia or even senile dementia—will force physicians to examine their older patients properly and accord them adequate medical care; this is essential if lives are to be saved from the terrible and total destruction that can result from unnecessary commitments to mental hospitals and last-stage nursing homes and neglect as "hopeless cases."

Take NIA Director Butler's own tale of the seventy-year-old single engineer who abruptly became confused and disoriented. He was so terrified by these feelings he wouldn't leave his room. Friends called a doctor who wouldn't come, insisting he could do nothing, that the man belonged in a nursing home or mental hospital, and it was only under pressure from neighbors that the physician finally did arrive, only to reiterate the same things. Fortunately the engineer was still capable of refusing this "medical" advice—but he did agree to enter a regular medical hospital. Within a week he was out and in fine condition: tests and examinations had shown he was simply the victim of a virus infection that responded promptly to the proper medical treatment!

So common is this sort of thing that Dr. Libow has felt the need to coin a new term—pseudo-senility—to call the medical profession's attention to this situation. Other than physicians' attitudes, however, the myths of senility do come from one very real source: brain disorders—dementias and other problems.

THE ORGANIC BRAIN SYNDROMES

Mental impairment can either be functional or organic: functional, as with J and R, mimics the myth of senility and is actually depression—as we shall see in Chapter 6, a very widespread problem among those over sixty-five. The other kind is the organic brain syndrome (OBS), which is defined by the American Psychiatric Association as a mental disturbance resulting from some impairment of the brain tissue itself.

OBS can be further broken down into "acute," and "chronic" conditions. If "acute," the problem is temporary and the condition reversible, as with the engineer described earlier. Acute OBS is the equivalent of Dr. Libow's "pseudo-senility," a condition due to some physical change or toxic manifestation that can be treated and cured. If "chronic," however, the brain damage is permanent and the condition irreversible.

If the cause is tracked down in time, any person with acute OBS can be restored to health, regardless of age, so it is imperative that the proper specific diagnosis be made at once. Demand it. Anything that interferes with the nourishment of the brain—the supply of oxygen and food (essentially glucose)—by the blood stream can produce acute OBS: including pneumonia, emphysema, heart conditions and arteriosclerosis (all of which interfere with either the blood supply or its oxygen content); malnutrition (a 1968 study found this present in at least 10 percent of older Americans); too much or too little thyroid hormone; abuse or simple misuse of drugs (see Chapter 8); kidney or liver conditions (cirrhosis or hepatitis); and much more. Dr. Butler has found more than one hundred causes of acute OBS, yet these can almost invariably be turned around with proper medical care. The danger is that, if they are neglected too long, they will eventually become irreversible and chronic, and a life will be unnecessarily ruined; the person condemned to a permanently demented state.

It is the chronic, permanent dementias that are so terrible.

THE DEMENTIAS

These devastating and even dehumanizing diseases have always been feared by mankind—it is the madness King Lear feared. One of the most tragic parts of the destructive myth of senility lies in the fact that many consider dementia and senility to be synonymous with old age, and so it is that the thought of the later years can stir up the paralyzing fear of losing one's mind and being "put away." It was to raise the shadow of this fear from the over-sixty-five person that this book was written.

The term "dementia" actually means a deterioration in intellectual or mental capacity and the condition may begin quite insidiously. The victim may at first even be able to continue his or her work at home or on the job, with any serious interference with functioning developing only slowly. The stricken doctor, for example, may be capable of handling his long-standing patients but no longer be able to come up with the less obvious diagnoses on new patients or the more complex prescriptions required. Loss of memory is often the first distinct symptom in this disturbing process.

Dr. Terry outlines the rest: "The earliest signs are usually related to impaired judgement and somewhat slowed thought processes. Recent memory then becomes defective. Speech disturbance is often quite early, with particularly frequent anomie, a difficulty in calling up nouns. Disorientation in time and place is common. Emotional disturbances and even delusions follow, with ultimate deterioration of personal habits, speech and total memory."

The most common of the dementias—some two-thirds of all cases—is Alzheimer's Disease, which can first appear as early as the forties. In fact, it was a fifty-one-year-old woman in 1902 whose disease, described by the German neurologist Alois Alzheimer, is now known to be the same as the disorder formerly termed senile dementia. The clinical symptoms do not differ materially from those of any of the other dementias, but the brain itself gradually atrophies, shrinks in both size and weight; a lessened cortex develops, with a marked loss of neurons and an increase in the size of the ventricles (spaces) of the brain. Pathologists also find, on microscopic examination of the brain following death, that there are an increase in "tangles" (twisted fibers in the neuron cell bodies) and in "plaques" (abnormal neuronal elements with dense central masses of a hard protein called amyloid).

The odd part of all this is that, as Dr. Terry points out: "There are quantitative differences but not qualitative ones between the brain of the normal aged person and that of those with Alzheimer's Disease." Just what this similarity means is still a mystery, but we will discuss the suspected causes after looking at the other forms of dementia.

Creutzfeldt-Jakob Disease is much less common than Alzheimer's and has a rapidly fatal course. From its onset, the degeneration of the cerebral cortex can be seen to progress literally from day to day until the disease's termination, commonly within a year. It is also unique among the dementias in that the cause is a so-called "slow virus," one that may be present in the body for as long as twenty or thirty years before it sets off obvious symptoms.

Huntington's Disease—a still rarer dementia—is best known for its most famous victim, Woody Guthrie, and is unique in that it is inherited as a defective gene. It starts quietly in the victim's thirties or forties, but proceeds steadily over a period of twelve to fifteen years until the victim's death, and is marked by a great loss of neurons, often in the cortex.

And, finally, there is Pick's Disease. Also a degenerative disease affecting the cerebral cortex, this one is so rare (it's barely one-fiftieth as common as Alzheimer's) that little is really known about it. It is sometimes genetic, but often there is no family history.

The Causes of Dementia

There are several theories about the cause of Alzheimer's Disease but the final proof of any one of them is still in the future, as is the relationship of this disorder to the normal changes that take place in the normally aging brain. For instance, there have been families that have shown a genetic distribution or inheritance of Alzheimer's similar to that in Huntington's. Reduced blood flow as a result of arteriosclerosis has also been suspected, but some think this is only an effect of the disease and not a cause. Then too, excessive amounts of aluminum have been found in the neurons of Alzheimer's victims and some investigators are looking into this phenomenon.

Evidence has come to light of late that points to the disease as a transmitted one. In 1976 the Nobel Prize in medicine was shared by Dr. D. Carleton Gajdusek of our National Institutes of Health for his work on a rare disease called Kuru (the Laughing Disease) that was destroying an obscure people in the remote hinterlands of New Guinea. He discovered the cause to be a new type of slow virus that also seems to be the cause of Creutzfeldt-Jakob Disease. Further proof for person-to-person transmission has come in the form of recent tragic deaths. In two of these—in New York City and in Europe—the disease was transmitted by the transplantation of corneas from people who were not known at the time to have died of the disease. In Switzerland, the disease was transmitted to two people as a result of electrodes implanted in their brains for diagnostic studies; these electrodes were found to have been used on a person who later died of the disease. One of these victims has died and the other was in a coma of more than three months' duration at the time of this writing. In addition, a neurosurgeon who had worked on patients with the disease died of it himself—indicating that self-inoculation is a danger to all those who actually handle or come in contact with diseased tissue. Yet a further piece of evidence is that it has been proved possible to innoculate a particular strain of mice with a specific strain of virus from a disease called scrapie and get brain changes strongly reminiscent of some of those in Alzheimer's.

Finally, the most recent suspected cause of Alzheimer's is a condition that doctors term autoimmune disease. In essence, the body's immune system, its defense mechanisms, turns on itself and attacks the body's own tissue (including the brain tissues). In a sense it develops a sort of allergy to the body's own proteins, a condition that seems to increase in incidence as the human being gets older. It is a theory that is being increasingly favored by many experts—but ultimately it is still a theory. For the present the real cause of the chief dementia—Alzheimer's Disease—is still a mystery.

HOW COMMON ARE THESE DEMENTIAS?

Again the picture is terribly confused. The myth of senility has given us the popular concept that almost all those who are old must suffer "senility"—yet nothing could be further from the truth. NIA Director Butler puts the figures for the dementias this way: "I suppose the best you can say is that it's possible that as many as maybe one million older Americans—an awfully rough guess—may have some form of intellectual dysfunction—but that's only one out of twenty-three. It's far less than the public's general image of what happens to people as they grow older." What troubles him is simply that "the data base is just not there to make even an *educated* guess."

The figures are confusing and one can almost pick one's own. Most commonly quoted are those given by Dr. David B. Tower, Director of the National Institute of Neurological and Communicative Disorders and Stroke: "Recent estimates indicate that in the Northern European population aged 65 years and older, the prevalence of severe dementia is 4.4 percent . . . mild to moderate dementia is 11 to 12 percent . . . At least two-thirds of the cases of severe senile dementia have classical Alzheimer's Disease."

Many experts suggest these figures are indicative of the extent of the disease in the United States as well but, on the other hand, we know that 5 percent or slightly less of all Americans over the age of sixty-five are in nursing homes—and the usual guess is that perhaps half of these have OBS. This gives us a figure of perhaps 2.5 percent rather than Dr. Tower's 4.4. And Dr. Adrian M. Ostfeld, Yale University professor of epidemiology and public health, says: "There are no accurate assessments of incidence or prevalence of either Alzheimer's Disease or senile brain disease [OBS] . . . It is therefore, well recognized that Alzheimer's Disease is rare. I am sure, also, that clinically detectable senile brain disease is much less prevalent than is commonly believed. Only about one-half percent of persons sixty-five and over are institutionalized and that includes institutionalization for all reasons. . . . [and]. . . . senile brain disease must account for a minority of institutionalized cases."

Drs. Kazuo Hasegawa and Akhide Karasawa of the Tokyo Metropolitan Institute for Gerontology and St. Marianna University have done a study that carries particular weight since it was done with government support. Their study, encompassing 5,000 Tokyo residents aged sixty-five and older living at home, found that of them all about 4.5 percent suffered from these dementias—33 percent with the severe form, 30 percent with the moderate, and 37 percent with the mild.

THE END TO SENILITY

So, as of right now, it is really impossible to say how many people suffer from *dementia*. What it is possible to say, however, is that none suffers from *senility*. There is just no such thing—if the medical profession would only listen to its own experts and recognize it. There is depression (which as we shall see is eminently and successfully treatable) and there are organic brain syndromes, some of which are also readily reversible by modern medical care. Even those that are not reversible can be vastly helped, as we shall explore in Chapter 9.

The major problem, as summed up in part by Dr. Bertram S. Brown, Director of the National Institute of Mental Health, is this: "Diagnoses of chronic organic brain syndromes are more indiscriminately formulated in the United States [than in England] and . . . aged psychiatric patients [those with depression] are more commonly characterized as brain impaired although evaluation of their cognitive status would suggest the presence of affective dysfunction [depression]. . . . *There is ample evidence to suggest that placement of the patient in inappropriate treatment facilities as a result of inaccurate diagnosis may have deleterious, and even fatal effects.*" [italics mine]

As a result of ignorance and indifference, many of our elderly are literally being driven into dementia, even killed. It is not only up to the physicians, but up to the public to call a halt to this practice. The public must declare, "No more senility!"

CHAPTER 3

The Truth About Memory in the Older Person

AFTER FORTY years of marriage, C knew her husband was upset as soon as he came home. His troubled remarks worried her too: "When I got to the supermarket, I couldn't remember what I'd gone there for. . . . Am I getting senile?" There was no hint of laughter in his voice and C tried to reassure him—"Oh, now you know you did the same thing when our first child was born. I sent you out for her formula and you came back without it"—but he looked at her for a few moments and said, "But I was thirty then and knew it was only forgetting—everybody does that, it was perfectly normal then. But now . . ."

He was right and he was wrong. When a young man forgets, he shrugs his shoulders and ignores it—but an older person's forgetfulness is perfectly normal too.

When it happens to him, however, he tends to worry about it because the senility myth is so strong. What is the truth about memory? Does it really fade as the years pass, does the person imperceptibly slip into a doddering, foggy old age? Here are the facts.

WHAT IS MEMORY?

Everyone knows what it is to remember; we do it all the time and never give it a thought. We pick up the phone and quickly dial as many as ten digits to call our home; we remember the faces of friends and relations and the people we deal with and the meanings of many tens of thousands of words; we remember the date of our birthday, how many minutes in the hour or days in the year, maybe even our own social security number. We recall enormous numbers of facts and experiences, some of which go back twenty or fifty or even a hundred years. As Dr. Bernard M. Patten, professor of neurology at the Baylor College of Medicine and a memory expert, points out, some people can recite the entire previous Sunday's sermon from memory, or the value of the mathematical symbol pi out to as many as three hundred and twenty-six places. This is actually "easier than you might think," he emphasizes. "For one thing, there's no such thing as a strain on the brain—a person can file an unlimited amount of information in his memory."

Exactly how this is done is not certain. Although a good deal is known about the mind, many things about it are still a mystery—and the precise neurological mechanism of memory is one of them. We do, however, possess many scattered bits and pieces of information about how this amazingly intricate system works, and how to make it work much more efficiently for us.

It's known, for example, that the hippocampi—a pair of bean-shaped structures buried roughly in the center of the brain under the cortex—are present in all mammals as well as in many other vertebrates. These structures are evidently essential for the permanent storage of memories (what is called long-term memory), for when they are diseased and must be removed, the patient can clearly remember events occurring before the operation—but nothing at all of what happens afterward for more than a few moments.

We also know that any experience we undergo is believed to leave a "trace," a mark or change of some sort in our neurons or brain tissue, but since we don't yet know exactly what this trace is—physical, physiological or chemical—scientists have not yet been able to track it down. Drs. Gary Lynch and Philip W. Landfield, psychobiologists at the University of California at Irvine, believe, however, that chemical agents of some kind are responsible, that their presence or absence, some sort of biochemical marking system, accounts for the programming of memories into neural circuits. According to this theory, a nerve impulse traveling over a particular neural pathway leaves a physical memory trace that promotes the passage of succeeding impulses or stimuli over the same route—and perhaps this is why we memorize things more easily by simply repeating them over and over again. It is a view supported by many neuroscientists.

Scientists have also discovered they can modify memory in experimental animals, chiefly in mice and rats, which are the most useful subjects because they can be taught certain tasks, such as how to run a maze, and remember them afterward. These experiments have implications for human beings as well, particularly for the older person. It has been found, for instance, that animals given electroconvulsive shocks strong enough to cause brain seizures or convulsions within a few hours of their training will suffer significant loss of memory, as will animals treated with anesthetics, such as ether and fluothane, or with barbiturates. The same thing will happen if the animal is deprived of that stage of sleep called REM, or rapid eye movement, during which the mind is alert and the body is sleeping—some researchers call it "paradoxical sleep."

On the other hand, stimulant chemicals such as strychnine or picrotoxin, as well as others, can actually *improve* memory when administered up to an hour after the animal's training. A similar improvement in memory occurs when the hippocampus is electrically stimulated by means of implanted electrodes.

Sometimes it has been possible to do limited experiments under special conditions on human brains as well. The famous Canadian neurosurgeon Dr. Wilder Penfield had occasion to expose the brains of more than 1100 patients while performing radical surgery for epilepsy. Since the brain tissue feels no pain, he was able to apply local anesthetics only, the kind your dentist uses for drilling, instead of putting the patients totally to sleep, and found that electrical stimulation of the brain at various points caused them to experience vivid recall of forgotten events, especially visual or auditory experiences. Dr. Penfield noted that, although he was stimulating the cortex itself with his electrodes, the actual memories came from the underlying hippocampi which, as he put it, "seem to store keys-of-access to the record of the stream of consciousness."

On the other hand, Dr. Karl S. Lashley, an American psychologist who pioneered in studies of the brain and learning, concluded from his own extensive studies that any particular piece of information may be stored in an extensive number and variety of neurons widely scattered throughout the brain rather than in any sharply localized group of neurons.

Is memory localized in the hippocampus? Is it spread out over a number of other areas of the brain as well? The controversy is a hot one, and the extreme complexity of the brain makes the debate difficult to resolve. Any final or definitive answer may be off somewhere in the twenty-first century, or conceivably even beyond that . . . but meanwhile there are some specific things we know about long- and short-term memory.

THE LONG AND THE SHORT OF IT: HOW *YOU* REMEMBER

A patient once told me: "My mother is in her nineties and she can remember things that happened seventy or eighty years ago—but not things that happened last week." This difference between the capacity for long-term memory (recall of the past) and short-term memory (recall of the present) may not be as great as has been believed, but there is no question that it plays a major role in what and how we recall.

In essence the process of memory consists of three elements: registration or storage; retention; and retrieval of information. When something is to be "remembered," your mind must register it somewhere in your brain (most likely in the hippocampus); it must be preserved (as the memory trace); and, finally, it must be kept in a form in which it can be brought back to consciousness as needed. There must also be some mechanism to allow for simple immediate use of such information or experiences as are needed only for the moment and which would never be used again even if they were committed to permanent retention. The human brain accomplishes all this through short-term and long-term memory.

Short-term memory is a sort of mental scratch pad. You jot down something for immediate reference—a phone number you intend to use only once, for instance—and then less than a minute later it can be forgotten. You might repeat the number a couple of times just to keep it in there a little longer, but once it is gone, it is gone for good.

But what if it's something to which you want to hold on? That's where long-term memory comes into play. You might repeat the number a couple more times or write it down to make it visual or use any of a dozen other tricks, but by the time you're through, that item of information will have been committed to permanent bulk storage. It is a fantastic system. Long-term memory contains (presumably in memory traces) all the records of our long years of experience and information—and this can be ninety or a hundred years or more. It has within it virtually everything that we have ever committed to memory, just sitting there waiting to be retrieved.

This does not always mean that the information is easy to retrieve, however. Looking for something in our short-term memory bank is relatively simple because there are a limited number of items to be checked, but the long-term memory contains a vast amount of stored material. That we can call things up at all is incredible considering the size of the task—and we are beginning to understand how it works. It has been shown, for example, that long-term memory for words is like a thesaurus with words of related meanings stored near each other. Once the word "dentist" is remembered, for instance, it is easier to remember the word "tooth." At the end of this chapter we'll have some tricks you can use for improving your memory.

WHAT DOES AGE REALLY DO TO ONE'S MEMORY?

The myth of senility has it that loss of memory is part and parcel of the whole process of degeneration and disintegration after the age of sixty-five. Like the rest of the myth, however, scientific studies have repeatedly shown this belief to be fiction and not fact.

Recently concluded studies of 153 people ranging in age from fifty to ninety-one, conducted by a team headed by University of Chicago professor of psychiatry Dr. Robert L. Kahn, revealed that their complaints of memory impairment did not jibe with their actual memory capability and objective performance. Strangely, those with very real memory loss (victims of organic brain syndrome) commonly minimized their loss. Dr. Kahn found that memory complaints had to be differentiated from actual memory performance, and that depression—a very widespread problem of older people—seemed to be at the bottom of many of the memory complaints where there was no actual impairment. It is well known that depression can actually interfere with memory—and we've already seen how depression mimics the stereotyped "senility."

But depression, Dr. Kahn found, also produced other side effects so that normal forgetfulness—failing to buy something at the store or misplacing one's eyeglasses or keys—that might be ignored by others was seen by the depressed person in particular as absolute proof of mental deterioration. Moreover, those people who complained the most about their memories were actually often found to have much better memories than those who did not complain and those who—like C's husband—merely become alarmed at a dramatic bit of forgetting. The depressed person will exaggerate such minor instances and complain frequently.

As for the commonly repeated platitude that recent memory in the elderly is much poorer than long-term: the hard fact is that almost all those Dr. Kahn studied proved to have higher scores for their memory of recent events than for their memory of remote ones!

Thus we see there is a lot of mythology about what the elderly can and cannot remember. There are a number of emotional factors, however, that do enter into the memory picture and distort recall. Depression obviously interferes with a person's feeling about his memory and can provoke considerable complaints, but society's attitudes and beliefs *prepare* the older person to find his memory failing and thus makes it a self-fulfilling prophecy. The elderly person may report failing memory even though it may actually be no different from what he or she had as a younger man or woman. Then, too, one's youth often seems a nicer time in our youth-oriented society, with its attitudes and rewards for the young. As a result it's more agreeable for many elderly people to contemplate their youths and so they "remember" long ago much better, recalling their triumphs and successes and "forgetting" the immediate present which lacks the bright excitement and thrills of the past. In short, one could say the elderly are rewarded for recalling the past and penalized for remembering the immediate present!

Moreover, the very methods for testing memory are suspect, for the older persons—particularly those in their seventies and eighties—come from a different and sometimes lesser educational background. As a result, the tests themselves, designed specifically to test today's youth, may penalize the older person. And then finally there is the very simple fact that all of us can forget—emotions do block certain names, memories can be misplaced. As long as the older person doesn't misinterpret this occurrence, as long as he views it not as a sign of "senility" or of mental deterioration but as a normal human problem, then there need *be* no problem.

Dr. Steven H. Zarit, a professor of gerontology and psychiatry at the University of Southern California, is working at techniques to improve the memory of older people. He and his colleagues have found it helpful for those concerned with their memories "to build their confidence in themselves and not to exaggerate instances where they forget things—this way they can be calmer when they forget what they went to the store for." As he points out: "Memory at any age is something you have to work at," and his research "seems to suggest that those who say they can remember the past better than the present have more concerns in their present life than they had in the past—the past may have been a better time in their lives."

He also finds that all the tricks people use to improve their memory work just as well for older people. Here are some of the classic ones.

IMPROVING YOUR MEMORY—TECHNIQUES THAT WORK

Memory expert Dr. B.M. Patten believes that "improving one's memory can be a lot of fun. All it takes is a little practice and a sense of humor." And the techniques we use are still very much like those originally invented by the ancient Greeks.

Most memory system historians point to Thessaly in 477 B.C. as the point of origin for memory techniques and a Greek poet—Simonides by name—who attended a wild shindig of his day, a banquet in the halls of the local nobleman, as the author. The poet left early after reciting his poem—just in time to escape the roof's collapse and the flattening of the nobleman and his guests beyond recognition. There was no record of those who had been there and officials asked Simonides to recall the names. At first he couldn't remember more than a very few, but then he discovered that by visualizing in his mind's eye the name and face of the person and the place where he sat at the table, he could quickly recall every single one. Out of this visualization he created a whole system of memory aids that the Greeks named for their goddess of memory—Mnemosyne—and today we still speak of these techniques as mnemonics. They're essentially a matter of associating a hard-to-recall object with another easy-to-remember one in whatever way is comfortable for the individual.

Cicero did it by nailing key points consecutively to the walls or furniture in his home so that by visualizing walking through his house room by room the items (the points to be covered in his oration, say, or the items in a long list) would be there for him to see in their proper order. Another technique is coding, as in the old trick of remembering how to set your clock for Daylight Saving Time by the phrase, "Spring forward—Fall back." Yet a third technique is to visualize a dramatic or absurd image in connection with the things to be remembered. I had to buy grapes, a loaf of bread, orange juice and tea yesterday: I thought for a few minutes and then visualized a big "T" blocking my door and not letting me out—or back in without the items. Then on one arm of the T, I hung a loaf of bread and on the other arm a can of frozen juice—but instead of orange juice pouring out of the can, I visualized large purple grapes! Sure, it's all a game but if you learn to play it you'll be amazed at how much you can depend on your memory.

When it comes to numbers, however, that's a different ball game, despite the feats of such as George Parker Bidder, a ten-year-old boy in the last century who had a forty-three digit number read to him backwards and then promptly repeated it exactly—in its correct order! In the *AMA Update* of Christmas 1972 (Volume 2/Number 10), Dr. Patten provided the following "MEMORY ALPHABET" to help people remember numbers by converting them into easily recalled words:

For this number . . .	Think of this letter and word	Memory Helps
1	t (ton)	The letter has one downward stroke
2	n (new)	The letter has two downward strokes
3	m (me)	The letter has three downward strokes
4	r (roar)	Fourth letter in "four"
5	l (live)	"L" is the Roman numeral for 50 (or 5 × 10)
6	d (Dix-ie)	Letter looks like a backward 6
7	k (boy's name Kevin)	Letter looks like two 7s joined together
	Also g, q, and hard c	g, q and hard c all have "K" sounds
8	b (bait);	script b has two loops like number 8
	also w (wait)	script w looks like an 8 lying down
9	p (pine) also f (fine)	Letter p looks like a backward 9; think of a man's pipe, which looks like a 9 with a puff of smoke (puff contains both letters) curling upward to form a 9
0	x (used with o in tic-tac-toe) s (so; also z (zero)	All three letters make a sound like a grindstone which is shaped like an 0

EXAMPLE: The memory alphabet letters for pi (3.1415) are M, T, R, T, and L.

Think of My TuRTLe.

We can now move ahead to something no one needs mnemonics to remember. . . .

CHAPTER 4

A New Level of Sexuality – New Possibilities for Sex in the Golden Years

APPROACHING SEX with some excitement and fresh thinking can produce new levels and experiences in sexuality in the later years. Repeated observations and studies have shown that the only real difference between the sexual responses and behavior of the younger and the older adult is one of quantity and not quality. With the greater differences and individuality among older people, the outlook can actually be brighter for distinctive and stimulating sexual patterns among the elderly rather than the monotony that so many young people complain of suffering in their sex lives. Certainly today's medically and psychologically healthier society, with its more rational view of sexuality and greater acceptance of personal differences and life styles, promises further opportunities for making old age obsolete and putting an end to "senility."

As one enters one's sixties, however, it is vital to have the knowledge and understanding necessary to anticipate and cope with the normal physiological changes that occur in one's normal sexual functioning. If one has such information, together with reasonably good health and an interested and interesting partner, then one can expect continued, pleasurable sexual relations—along with other essential physical and emotional satisfactions—virtually as long as life itself continues. Age is no barrier to sex—although there is likely to be a reduction in the patterns and amount of sexual activity just as there is with physical activity generally. As with any activity, the amount and the degree of participation in later life would seem to depend largely on the lifelong patterns that have prevailed—the greater the activity in young adulthood the more there will be in the later years of life. Not only can sexual intercourse continue into the nineties but for some the frequency of sex even increases in the very late years.

Those factors that actually make sexual activity grind to a halt as people pass the mythical milestones of sixty ("the big six," as it's often termed, indicating its powerful and emotionally threatening nature) and sixty-five (when retirement fuses with birthday) are to a very large degree due to the destructive attitudes of society, which the unprepared person converts into self-fulfilling prophecies. Strangely, in the midst of the current sexual revolution that has freed our young people, their grandparents still find themselves locked into the patterns of the past, a sort of medical and social version of the Dark Ages bounded by taboos. This is the time for older Americans to assert their own rights to a healthier emotional and sexual life style—and there is evidence this is happening.

This chapter presents the information needed to achieve that end, to prevent the secondary impotence that threatens the sexually innocent and ignorant, to dispel the myths, to make the sexual lives of older people richer and more fulfilling, to deal with both the normal changes of time and with the results of operations and diseases, to open new possibilities.

SEX IN THE ELDERLY: THE TABOOS, THE MYTHS—AND THE FACTS

To understand the problem one must comprehend something about the deep-rooted, irrational nature of taboo. The word itself comes from the Polynesian *tabu* which means prohibited or forbidden, but also carries with it many underlying complexities. It is an ambivalent concept, including something of both the magical and the sacred, the pure and the impure, the holy and the dangerous, with implications of power, peril, and even a sense of being unclean. So it is that when behavioral scientists speak of the taboo against sex among the elderly they include a whole range of feelings whose intensity makes investigations difficult and puts into question the individual's or society's rational handling of the subject. It is this taboo that makes it hard for the elderly to enjoy their sexuality as fully and openly as they would like.

The taboo nature of sex among the elderly also confuses matters when the older person wants information or help for sexual problems from his doctor. In fact, experts in human sexuality find many, if not most, doctors still hesitant and uncomfortable about asking patients in general, and older ones in particular, about their sexual relations, even though this is a medically legitimate and important part of their initial interview with a patient. While many of the elderly do resent such inquiries, many others welcome the opportunity to discuss such questions and seek sex help and advice when they are given the chance.

The exact reason for this taboo is not fully clear but experts see a number of factors responsible. The actuality that it has survived our current sexual revolution is evidence that the taboo goes much deeper and is far stronger than most of our attitudes toward sex left over from the Victorian Era. The children of today's elders—even though they may themselves be sexually liberated—are acutely uncomfortable and may object vigorously when the subject of their parents' sexual relations is brought up. Trained observers suspect this reaction may arise from the incest taboo—one is not allowed to equate parents with sex—or from oedipal feelings, an early attachment of a child to the parent of the opposite sex, with attendant hostility toward the other.

Then too there is the vestige of the American attitude that still somehow clings to the Puritan notion that sex should be engaged in primarily for procreative reasons and only secondarily for recreation. The elderly have had their children. Much of the rest of the world looks upon sex as play—while Americans even work at having fun—but even there our older citizens are not supposed to play at things, because "it's not dignified."

There is, in addition, a whole set of myths about normal sexual behavior that joins with the prejudices and stereotypes of ageism to contribute to a general desexualization of the elderly. The result, as Dr. Butler sees it: "Derision, denial and despair have been our primitive responses to sexuality in old age, due to misinformation, misapprehension, and a general prejudice against the old . . . Many people, young and old, are astonished or embarrassed at the idea of human beings making love in their seventies, eighties and even beyond." Out of such reactions have arisen the many so-called jokes about the sexual behavior and capacity of the aged; the remarks that someone is "too old for such nonsense," "all dried up," "fading fast"; and the attitudes that cause elderly men and women who are interested in dating or even marrying to be repeatedly warned, "Don't make fools of yourselves." Dr. Martin Leshner, a psychologist at Indiana University-Purdue University, tells of the sixty-year-old man who on his remarriage was given with great jocularity, a case of spray starch as a wedding gift. His new wife frankly assured them he had no need for the present.

Let's look at the mistaken concepts behind such a gift.

The "over the hill" mythology implies that between the ages of sixty and sixty-five the sexual decline finally hits bottom and sexuality is over. The reality, however, is that the ability to enjoy sex remains throughout life.

Another damaging myth is that of "fragility"—sexual activity is dangerous because the old are just too physically delicate. This can lead to an actual fear of broken bones from sexual intercourse (which is sheer nonsense unless there is some serious and specific disease present) or of heart attacks (actual studies, as we'll soon see, show a very low frequency). In fact, estimates are that the effort of sexual intercourse is roughly equivalent only to that of walking up two flights of stairs.

Then, too, there is the assumption that only the young are beautiful and sexually arousing. Sexual attractiveness can come from many sources—character, charm, facial expressions, body movements—but a man's potbelly or unshaven face are not attractive at any age, nor is a dirty or unkempt woman. The older person—no less than the younger—must put some effort and thought into making himself or herself sexually attractive, but having done so, there is frankly no reason why he or she can't be appealing.

The "dried-up juices" myth probably arose from the idea that the sexual juices literally dry up, that the man can no longer produce semen nor the woman vaginal lubrication. While both secretions are somewhat reduced, as we shall see, neither change actually presents any problems for those older people who keep up an active sex life.

The "neuter woman" canard says that the older woman has no sexual interest at all—and when she does show a normal interest in sex she is looked upon as representative of another stereotype, the "depraved woman." All of this leaves the older woman in a terrible bind, but fortunately, with women's liberation, women are being freed. As Dr. Nancy Datan, a psychologist at the University of West Virginia, put it in a presentation before the 1977 Annual Convention of the American Psychological Association, in the future we may hope to see "The Emergence of the Sensuous Grandmother."

One hopes that, with the exposure of many of these myths and of ageism itself, a new understanding and honesty will permit us to bury these destructive myths and allow both women and men a new freedom to express their essential sexuality. Some are already leading the way: the sports car of a Californian in his seventies features a bumper sticker reading "I'm not a dirty old man—I'm a sexy senior citizen."

Cultural influences, however, produce such intense pressure on the members of a society that they can provoke self-destructive thinking and behavior. The older American too often accepts our ageism with its negative sexual attitudes and, overwhelmed by its unlovely picture of both older people and their sexuality, literally gives up without trying. The result is a self-fulfilling prophecy: any attempts at sexual relations inevitably end in disaster. When older people permit their sexual desires to surface they may see them as shameful and so avoid any opportunities for sexual encounters—yet the reality is that sexuality can and does continue for men and women into their nineties.

THE FEAR OF FAILURE

There is one overriding fear that can damage sexuality, however. It is particularly important since our culture puts such a heavy overemphasis on success and performance. The man tends to equate his sexual potency with masculinity and the first evidence of any change in sexual patterns strikes fear into his heart; the woman on the other hand is more inclined to fear the loss of physical attractiveness—although, with women's liberation and the new sexual climate, there is considerable likelihood that older women may soon show more concern and anxiety over their orgasmic capacity.

In both sexes, a problem that psychologists refer to as

"spectatoring" is likely to intervene. When the man senses any reason to question his ability to function sexually (usually the normal physiological changes, but they may cause him to feel "it's all over now"), he ceases to become a partner and participant in the ongoing behavior of the sexual act. Instead of experiencing and enjoying the stimulation of sex play, he begins to watch himself, checking for the presence or appearance of each feeling and reaction; he becomes a spectator in the stands critically evaluating the procedure and the reactions of the players (specifically himself).

The result, of course, is sheer disaster. This spectatoring attitude prevents or cuts off the communication with his own body and his own feelings that seem to be a necessity for erection. It is a pattern that can appear at any age, but it occurs especially in the man who has entered or passed through the sixties—and one who goes along with the cultural attitude that he is "aging" and coming to the end of his sexual life. Spectatoring is particularly likely to occur, too, if a man has abstained from sex for some time for whatever reason.

Nor is spectatoring an exclusively male problem, for women may suffer from it as they too develop fears of their own performance. While the woman doesn't have the same need for a positive action like an erection in order to have sex, she does need to have her glands supply proper lubrication for the sex act—and this lubrication is the physiological equivalent of the male erection. As a result, fears about performance and the resultant spectatoring can lead to a failure as bad as a man's. If the lubrication fails, the sex act itself can cause her considerable pain (dyspareunia), and this in turn reduces any desire for sex and brings the additional fear of pain into play.

To further complicate matters, depression, too, often leads to a reduction of sexual activity in women; while, in the man, sexual dysfunction may lead to depression. However, since satisfactory sexual activity produces feelings of well-being, happiness, and self-worth—the very feelings needed to supply the emotions lacking in depression—sex may actually help to turn around this emotional problem.

As long as men and women avoid the fear that sexual changes signify "the end of everything," a ringing down of the curtain on their sex life, they can accept their physiologic changes with equanimity and go on to enjoy a rich and diversified sex life through the rest of their life span. But the key to their future is knowledge.

WHAT HAPPENS TO THE SEXUALITY OF THE MAN AS HE AGES

There really is no age limit to sexual activity in the normal healthy man and there are even those who only first develop their sexual capacities late in life. Havelock Ellis, the physician whose writing in the late nineteenth and early twentieth centuries first helped to break the conspiracy of silence thrown up around human sexuality, resolved his own lifelong impotency only when he was in his sixties. Dr. Harry J. Johnson, chairman of the medical board of the Life Extension Institute, recalls an eighty-one-year-old patient whose wife had recently died and who found that much as he missed her—what he missed most was their regular weekly sex. It is in the awareness of coming sexual changes and what they mean that the secret lies to successful sexuality in the later years.

In general, the man over sixty (and perhaps even over fifty as well) can expect that it will take him more time to achieve full penile erection, that this may not be as full or as firm as in his twenties and may not even be complete until just before ejaculation. The big danger is that since this is likely to be the first sexual change that he notices, the man may panic. Appalled, he may suddenly become convinced his sex life is nearly finished and feel less of a man: he may then begin to find excuses for avoiding sex with his spouse, thus arousing *her* feelings of being unattractive, stirring up all her negative feelings about herself (buttressed by society's myths). Should she now press him at this vulnerable time he may readily develop impotency, simply as a result of this misunderstood physiologic change, and major sexual problems could arise for both partners—and ultimately major marital problems as well.

Actually, if a man is capable of having an erection at *any* time (the evening, the morning, whenever) he is probably capable of satisfactory sexual activity. In fact, Masters and Johnson believe that aging *never* costs the ability to have an erection—that when this happens, psychological and not physiological causes should be sought, regardless of age.

Ejaculation, too, changes and may be of shorter duration, with decreased power, fewer expulsive contractions and less seminal fluid. Once the ejaculation has occurred, the erection subsides very rapidly and the man may not respond to sexual stimulation for a longer period than in the past—perhaps up to as much as several days. Moreover, ejaculation may not occur with every sexual act—and both partners must realize that ejaculation is not necessary for them to achieve both pleasure and satisfaction. Sometimes, too, the older man may even experience what doctors call "retrograde ejaculation"—the semen forced back into the bladder instead of out through the head of the penis.

Sexual satisfaction, however, is not to be judged by the performance level of the twenty-five-year-old (although in our youth-oriented society it sometimes seems that everything is evaluated by comparing it to the young). The pleasures of older, more mature sexuality come from a deep enjoyment of the relationship between a man and a woman: touching, caressing, and holding become more important and give enormous sensual satisfaction. Freud never said that sexuality was limited to the genitals. As one gets older, an important and even vital sense of well-being arises out of the pleasures and satisfactions derived from the acceptance and affection of a close marital and sexual relationship. In fact, experts seem to feel that having a partner is essential to survival—perhaps because of the emotional involvement, or simply because it means that you have someone to care for you.

Repeatedly, investigators in human sexuality find that the best way for both men and women to retain their sexual capacities and effectiveness is simply to continue their sexual functioning on a regular basis. Which brings us to the other side of the coin. . . .

WHAT HAPPENS TO THE SEXUALITY OF THE WOMAN AS SHE AGES

The vaginal lubrication process—the female physiologic counterpart of the male's erection—will similarly be affected with age. Not only does it take the older woman longer to achieve vaginal lubrication from the time actual sexual stimulation begins but the lubrication itself is not as copious as it was during youth. Furthermore, the vagina in the older woman tends to have less expansile capacity; with an actual loss in length, width, and elasticity—and the clitoris itself is reduced in size although there is no change in its sensitivity or its functioning.

Orgasm in the older woman usually lasts a shorter time and has less intensity but this does not reduce the pleasure of the sexual act. In younger women the uterus contracts rhythmically during orgasm in a manner very much like the contractions of the first stage of labor; however the older woman may suffer actual muscle spasms of the uterus during orgasm for as much as a minute and a half to two minutes and this may cause sudden severe lower abdominal pain and even considerable post-coital discomfort.

There was a time when hormonal or estrogen replacement was widely used to help the thinning out of the vaginal lining which can lead to pain during intercourse, but the current concern over the possible role of estrogen in certain tumors has made many physicians hesitant to prescribe it until its medical status is clarified. Most advise now that no woman continue taking an old prescription for hormones without checking first with her doctor.

An older woman may gradually lose virtually all her lubrication capacity and suffer a wasting and shrinkage of the vaginal lining tissues so that the occasional sexual act may prove both irritating and painful, but the many women who continue to lead active sex lives often suffer no difficulties even without hormonal assistance. Clearly the answer for both men and women is to maintain active and regular sexual activity, either with others or by themselves. Many experts suggest the value of self-stimulation or masturbation for the aged since they are so often widowed or alone.

WHAT ILLNESS OR SURGERY CAN DO TO SEXUAL ACTIVITY IN THE ELDERLY

However, another situation arises. Diseases, and operations in particular, invariably produce emotional reactions of all sorts and intensities, depending on the kind of illness or operation and the age of the sufferer. Those past sixty-five—already struggling with the emotional problems and depressions that come with age (as we'll probe more fully in our next chapter)—are distressed by sickness or surgery more than younger people. Any emotionally disturbing situation is likely to affect sexual patterns—but there are some disorders that are particularly hazardous in this respect and our culture's misconceptions of the older person worsen matters considerably.

Obviously any surgery that directly affects the genitourinary system (the sexual and urinary system, its organs and tissues) is especially disturbing to men, with its direct threat of genital mutilation or loss. (In women, the two systems are separate.) Thus prostate surgery (the prostate gland supplies the bulk of the seminal discharge) can be expected to produce a severe reaction. The most common prostate problem is a noncancerous overgrowth and it is most often treated simply by reaming the excessive tissue out so that it no longer interferes with urination. Sometimes, however, the prostate gland is removed by more extensive surgery either through an incision in the lower abdomen or—most radical and least often used—through an incision in the anal area. Only in this last form of surgery is there any serious physical threat of impotency. Investigators have shown that with proper presurgery explanations of the procedures, sex life is not affected and that 80 percent or more of patients retain their potency. Impotency is far more common, however, when cancer is present and radical extensive surgery performed. Much of the effect on the older patient, however, depends on the treatment and the person; the doctor is the one to advise on the future effects on sex of such surgery.

Kidney or bladder surgery is also threatening, but there are some indications that not the physical condition, but the presence of a willing sex partner, is the most important factor in retaining the man's potency after this kind of disease.

Heart attacks—"coronaries"—are one of the great sources of health fears among Americans, the men fearing for themselves and the women for their men. As a result, both the victim of the heart attack and his mate are concerned about the resumption of sex and its effect. As we've seen, sex isn't all that strenuous and is commonly well within the capacity of the average fully recovered victim of a heart attack; but one of the problems is that the couple—particularly when they are past sixty-five—have difficulty in getting the needed advice and information from their physician about when and how sexual relations should be resumed. And such resumption should only be done after medical consultation. There are two reasons for this problem. First, not too many physicians really know the answer and, second, most older patients—plagued by our taboos and cultural myths—hesitate to ask. Those who do, commonly get answers such as the one a seventy-eight-year-old man told me his doctor gave him: "Forget it—you have more important things to worry about." Not surprisingly, this makes the older person reluctant to ask the questions he (and she) needs most to be answered.

The myths proliferate where sex and coronaries are concerned. The "coital coronary," for example, is one of the great traditional fears—but clearly more myth than reality. Of course the doctor's advice must be the final arbiter of the amount of strain the coronary patient can bear, and it may even be necessary to consult a cardiologist to get the needed information, since physicians are often not that knowledgeable about the relationship between sexual intercourse and the heart.

Too, sexual intercourse is not the only strain that can precipitate a heart-attack death—masturbation is also said to be capable of causing this. And then, doctors have been known to tell their patients it's all right to have sexual relations—but only with their wives because they don't want the patient to get too excited. This may sound odd, but the statistics actually bear it out. A recent study of people with heart conditions who died as a result of intercourse showed that twenty-seven out of thirty-four were involved in extramarital relations in strange surroundings.

But how much of a risk is there really in sex? There has actually been one large-scale study done, in the early 1960s in Japan. It showed that of nearly 6,000 sudden deaths from heart disease, only eighteen were the result of sexual intercourse and these followed drinking alcohol and eating rich foods. Obviously there isn't all that much for the heart patient to fear from sex—especially if he sticks to his own wife. This *must be* a medical decision, however, that only a skilled and wise doctor can make. For those who suffer angina pectoris, for example, he might prescribe premedication; by eliminating both the fear and the presence of pain the sex would be made more enjoyable.

He may also advise a period following a heart attack—two or three months, or perhaps more—during which sexual relations may have to be avoided. Afterward the doctor may suggest having sex in a side-by-side position or even with the woman on top in order to reduce the stress on the coronary patient. In fact, Dr. Butler points out that self-stimulation might even start before intercourse and be a good way to initiate the resumption of sexual activity.

The NIA Director also tells of a woman and her husband in their seventies who were faced with the problem that the man had a severely damaged heart; they were very much in love and both desired sex together. Because their love meant so much to them, they decided together to continue their lovemaking with full awareness of the risk. Eventually he had a heart attack while they were making love and died in her arms. With such a free and full-knowing choice on both their parts, the wife was able to accept her painful loss. However the fear of such an attack that ordinarily haunts both husband and wife in such a situation can be a very difficult thing for a marriage to deal with. Psychological support may be necessary.

Strokes, too, introduce both physical and emotional problems with sex. The victim of this disease may well be frightened, but here again the services of a knowing physician is invaluable. He can inform the stroke patient whether sex is safe and, if so, that it will not precipitate another stroke. Then he can help and advise about the sex act itself if there are physical problems such as paralysis. Additionally, it is possible, even urged by many experts, for many paraplegics to have sexual relations with a partner in a variety of ways. There are experts in a specialty called rehabilitation medicine who are interested and knowledgeable in this area today and the family doctor can refer the person or couple to such professionals.

Diabetes, too, is a disease common in the elderly and it can cause impotency in men. Medical help is the essential element here, for many times the potency can be restored when the diabetes is properly controlled. It is well to remember that there are specialists in diabetes—diabetologists—who can be consulted when the family doctor has difficulty in handling and controlling this disorder.

Any effects of hysterectomy—the removal of the uterus—on sex in the older woman are usually not physical after a month or so of healing. However, this operation can have a strong emotional impact, for it is the removal of a part of a woman's sexual and childbearing system. Under such circumstances, expert help may be called for: either discussion with a particularly understanding gynecologist or family doctor, or help from a psychologist or psychiatrist.

More damaging—and more difficult to adjust to emotionally—is mastectomy or breast removal. This can have marked effects both on how the woman feels about herself and on how her husband feels. Both husband and wife may need time to adjust to this new situation. Conversations with other women who have suffered the same experience can often help patients, and the Reach to Recovery program of the American Cancer Society can provide a good deal of help, together with reading material. Local units of the American Cancer Society have information on this valuable rehabilitation program.

In the case of any of these disorders or operations, however, the husband or wife or both may fail to get over their initial negative feelings about the situation. In those instances, skilled professional help is definitely needed and should be sought immediately. The family doctor can usually steer the involved people to a competent psychologist or psychiatrist for necessary help or psychotherapy.

DEALING WITH MEDICAL PROBLEMS AND SEX

Dr. Leshner has found that loss of sexual functioning due to actual physical disabilities occurs less than is commonly assumed. It is possible, with expert advice and help, for many people who have suffered spinal injuries—paraplegics, even quadriplegics—to achieve satisfactory marital sex lives. There are professionals in many major rehabilitation centers who are specially interested in such problems and can help families—husbands and wives together—to find satisfying answers where there is love and a mutual desire to overcome this barrier to sex.

Fortunately there are not too many who find themselves in so extreme a situation. Far more common are those older people who have relatively minor sex problems and can either search out the answers for themselves—using some of the ideas here—or at least use these approaches to get the answers from a doctor.

SEX AND ARTHRITIS

Most common, of course, are the arthritic problems, for virtually everyone past the age of sixty (some 97 percent) has arthritis to an extent that can be seen on x-rays. Fortunately for most, it's a matter of limited difficulty—some pain now and again, or morning stiffness—but for at least ten million, chiefly among those over sixty or sixty-five, this arthritis (the kind called osteoarthritis) is severe enough to cause them problems with daily life. And when it gets bad enough, it can take a terrible toll on human sexuality.

As Dr. Richard Rogal, clinical psychologist of Los Angeles' Ranchos Amigos Hospital, puts it: "Arthritis often acts like a counteraphrodisiac." The effects can be surprisingly far-reaching. Janice B. Onder, a medical social worker, explains: "When a man feels he is causing pain to a woman he cares about, impotency within the relationship or seeking new sexual partners are possible."

Solving the sexual problems of the arthritic or other physically disabled person can sometimes be surprisingly simple. Here are a few aids a sufferer can use or ask his or her doctor about. For example, medication can be adapted to making sexual activity possible and enjoyable. Simply by working out the proper time interval between taking his regular medication and having sex, the arthritic can assure maximum freedom from pain during sex. Or the doctor can suggest some extra medication or even prescribe a special drug to be taken in advance.

Muscle relaxation may also help an arthritic in relieving pain during the day. Commonly this consists of such simple measures as soaking in a hot tub, applying heat locally to painful muscles or joints (with hot compresses or an electric heating pad), or a variety of limbering-up exercises. Using such techniques before sexual activity may make the difference between a happy sex life and none at all. Two other things to be considered are simply noting the time of day when the condition is least troublesome and planning sex activity for that time, and, finally, accepting the form of sexual activity that will cause least discomfort. There is a lot to choose among.

SOLVING THE PROBLEMS: THE WAYS OF SEX

With the freedom and flexibility resulting from today's sexual revolution, it is possible to get around most problems. The arthritic, for instance, can feel free to have sex at any time of day and he knows that there is no such thing as "normal" sex; any sexual activity that participating partners enjoy together is normal. Americans today are constantly exploring new dimensions in sex and there is no reason for the elderly not to exploit this new freedom and enjoy their sexuality.

Experts in human sexuality all urge that the older person explore totally new patterns and question the old. The retiree is free to have sex at any time of the day or night; the house is free of children. If the older person finds a particular time at which he or she is at his or her most energetic—that fact should be exploited to make sex fresh, new and exciting. New places should be tried for lovemaking, as well as new times and positions. Older partners have time to experiment in how to please each other; many of them have, over the years, gradually made lovemaking a mechanical matter. Now is the time to change and learn. In fact, older women may have their first chance to experience orgasm if the man will take his time and seek to learn what pleases his mate.

New coital positions or ideas can be found in the innumerable books on the market today—or the imagination may be quite enough if the older couple will only feel free to give up the "missionary" position. Stimulation of other erotic body areas is enjoyable and orgasms can be reached by hand or by oral-genital sex (which today is commonly practised and widely accepted). Frank discussion of sex with one's husband or wife can be both revealing and exciting as well. Older people have earned their fun—why should youngsters be the only ones to have it? The key of course is freedom, and the woman can take an active role in it as well as the man.

DRUGS, NOSTRUMS, APHRODISIACS—FOR AND AGAINST SEX

There is one more problem area with sex. As we will see later (in Chapter 8), the elderly are particularly susceptible to drugs and are more likely to overreact or to react adversely than younger people. Impotency in the man is often the price paid for the help of some of that vast array of powerful drugs that doctors use to make life healthier and longer. For example, the steroids (sometimes used for severe arthritis and other problems) are capable of inducing impotency—as are many of the drugs used for such disorders as heart conditions or high blood pressure (hypertension) and many others.

Should impotency suddenly appear in a man who has never had this problem before but is taking medication on the orders of his physician (or even some he has purchased himself in the drug store), it is wise to consult the doctor promptly. The change may simply be a reaction to some of the medication and be reversible by immediate action. Some of the strong, or even mild, tranquilizers, for example, can cause impotency while others (such as the phenothiazines, used as powerful tranquilizers, or other drugs used for hypertension) may produce an inability to ejaculate even though erections are not affected; while still other drugs prevent erections only. And in the woman, any tranquilizer, even the mild ones like Librium, can produce a depressive effect on her sexual feelings, as can antidepressant drugs such as Tofranil.

The effects of drugs on sexual feelings and/or performance, however, is something to discuss with one's physician because he can usually change the dosage or switch to an alternative medication while giving his patient the same protection. This, too, is why it is important to have a physician who is knowledgeable about the special medical requirements of the older person.

Certain very common causes of impotency are often missed by the older person. The man has a little too much to drink during a night out or perhaps at a family affair. The couple wants to make love—and the man suddenly finds himself impotent, perhaps for the first time. Panic sets in, particularly in the older man. He waits a day or two, prepares for sex—and then slips out to the kitchen for a quick drink or two to give himself a little courage or

[illegible] appens all over again!
[illegible] becomes overwhelm-
[illegible] doctor may even keep
[illegible] end a perfectly normal
[illegible] or, the physician taking
[illegible] "Next time you want
[illegible] impotency would be
[illegible] hol commonly has this
[illegible] call, Shakespeare once
[illegible] vith lechery—it giveth
[illegible] rformance"), and toler-
[illegible] ge. However, even bar-
[illegible] lved—so anything one
[illegible] nce arises.

[illegible] oted as saying, "There's
[illegible] a crook every hour to
[illegible] would seem true, for
[illegible] ose for quacks and
[illegible] one costs the United
[illegible] a year—and our older
[illegible] n group. Among the favorite nostrums perennially peddled are those for preventing or curing impotence—or for restoring sexual youth. The older person shouldn't trust anyone or anything that promises or guarantees results in the medical area. A good family doctor is an excellent protection, because a phone call will bring quick information on the value or legitimacy of such claims.

Aphrodisiacs have excited man's interest since time

immemorial—and have never really worked as promised. No drugs should be used by an older person without checking with his doctor first because of the especial danger of drug reactions, and aphrodisiacs are no exception (particularly since some, such as Spanish fly, can even kill). If the older person really wants aphrodisiacs, he or she might try the best of all and the most effective still—as recommended by the Kinsey investigators—good health, adequate sleep, proper exercise, and an interested partner, and, perhaps we should add, an *interesting* partner as well.

HOW DO YOU FIND THE RIGHT DOCTOR—OR THE RIGHT SEX THERAPIST?

The man or woman's loss of interest in sex or his development of impotency or other sexual impairments can involve a number of factors, such as boredom or fatigue, overeating or excessive drinking, medical or psychiatric disabilities—it has been estimated that as much as 90 percent of chronic impotence actually has a psychological cause. To pin down the cause of sex difficulties, however, the individual needs good medical advice and care, or the help of the new sex therapies.

Finding the right physician is not easy and is so big a subject with so many ramifications that we will defer it to Chapter 6. However, getting help for sexual problems may warrant an expert. When the older person gets his first examination by a new doctor, he or she will be able to tell whether this professional can be turned to for sex advice. If the doctor takes a sexual history as part of his routine medical history and asks frankly about current sexual activity and patterns in a way that shows he is comfortable talking about the subject—and makes the older person feel this way too—then he is someone that can be relied on.

If he is uncomfortable with human sexuality, as is still true of the majority of physicians today, one alternative is to call the nearest medical school. Courses on human sexuality are being given in increasing numbers today, and the school could give the names of those who teach such a course and also practice locally. It's always best to select a university-based medical school—Harvard or the University of Michigan or Stanford, for instance; the larger the school, too, the more likely they are to be giving such a course.

In this burgeoning area, however, there is a tragically large amount of quackery today and people have to be extremely careful. Masters and Johnson themselves have repeatedly expressed concern over the situation. In a recent seminar on the future of sex therapy, Dr. Masters warned that the public was being bilked—of 3,500 to 5,000 sex therapy clinics in the United States in 1974 not fifty could be considered legitimate! Medical interest will certainly increase the number of legitimate sex therapy clinics, but the chance for big money (a course of treatment can run a couple of thousand dollars or more), together with ready customers and an unstructured field that demands no specific training, qualifications, examinations, certification, or licensing, all combine to attract unscrupulous figures into the field. Here again, a call to a university medical school or teaching hospital may provide appropriate references or credentials.

The safest way for the serious person or couple to seek

help for sexual problems is to discuss them with a knowledgeable family doctor or psychotherapist, but if more special assistance is needed, a sex therapist may be the answer.

A NEW LEVEL OF SEXUALITY

That the older person is capable of sex is now obvious—scientific studies have even revealed a ninety-six-year-old man still capable of having erections. Moreover, since ejaculation has changed in the older man, he can control it better, even preserve his erection longer, so that he is capable of longer lovemaking before ejaculation brings it to a close.

All this is the quantitative side of sex, however, the physical side that is emphasized in youth and young adulthood, often to the neglect of the qualitative aspects: the caressing, the touching, the tenderness. Furthermore, a lifetime of lovemaking between husband and wife permits the acquisition of new insights and levels of relationships, of emotions and feelings, of ties that can only be found over decades of closeness. Aging is not just an ending or tapering off of life, but a development period just as adolescence or young adulthood are—and developmental for sexuality as well.

If we see human sexuality in its true light, as the epitome of human closeness and affection, and not simply as some mechanical act, a testing of something new and untried, then the later years become an ideal time to discover new heights. In these later years, the pressures of child-bearing and raising, the drive for success and material acquisitions, have all subsided and there is more time available for self, and for developing a mutual intimacy, a deeper, richer understanding of one another. And what better way than through the medium of sexuality.

With this new dimension, Rabbi Ben Ezra's words "Grow old along with me. . . ." become truly not a threat but an invitation!

CHAPTER 5

Mental Health and Emotional Problems: What to Do

DR. FRANCIS J. Braceland—one of America's great pioneers in geropsychiatry, former Psychiatrist-in-Chief of Hartford's Institute of Living and Chief of Psychiatry at Mayo Clinic—has been interested in the emotional problems of the aged for nearly half a century. He recalls how, when only a young resident, "I diagnosed a confused and depressed lady as senile simply because she was over sixty-five years of age . . . [and] . . . prepared her family for a chronic illness and a dim future. The lady recovered completely in about two weeks and left the hospital, and I have never gotten over that incident . . . I learned the hard way that impairment of a functional nature is not an uncommon happening in the elderly and that it responds to treatment then as it does in other periods of life." In short, he put his own end to "senility."

Of course there are those who suffer true organic brain

changes, as we discussed in Chapter 2. But then what are we to make of this fact, discovered during autopsies: the brains of many people diagnosed as "senile" from their behavior have shown few of the neurologic changes associated with the dementias—while the brains of others who have held important jobs right up to their deaths have been shown to contain severe brain pathology! Dr. Braceland offers an explanation, drawn from his long experience, for these seemingly contradictory facts: "The trouble with many individuals who exhibit senile behavior may be that they have 'quit,' have 'given up.' They have failed for some reasons, recognized or unrecognized, even by themselves, to stay in the main stream of daily life."

In short, by achieving an improved mental health and keeping up an active life the aging person can find help to put an end to "senility." For much of what doctors still all too quickly term "senility" is simply poor mental health, those emotional disturbances that all human beings are heir to but which may appear in somewhat different forms in those of different ages—just as various age groups may respond differently to physical illnesses, diseases, even to identical dosages of the same medications.

In this chapter we will examine what mental health is, how common emotional problems can be in the Third Age; what the warning signs are; what the nature of these problems is; and how they can either be prevented or treated.

WHAT *IS* MENTAL HEALTH?

All too often "mental health" is spoken of with that same vague reverence with which we mention motherhood, the flag, and religion, and its real meaning becomes lost in a welter of uncertain meanings. Perhaps the best way to explain it—since it cannot be defined as precisely as a mathematical formula or a strep throat—is to turn to the ways National Institute of Mental Health experts regard it. Mental health, they agree, is in a broad sense the way a person adjusts to life: it has to do with his ability to stay on top both of his life and of what is going on in the world around him, even when that going gets very rough. In short, good mental health involves a person's total emotional and behavioral life—the way he thinks, the way he acts, and his relationships with others.

Obviously no one can pass through life entirely without worries, anxieties, or depressions. Things happen to us all the time that can provoke anger, anxiety, depression, fear, distrust, and the like. An outstanding characteristic of mental health, however, is that these very reactions—anger, depression, and the rest—are only temporary passing emotions, feelings that are never allowed to become part of the individual's ongoing reactions to every detail of his or her day-by-day life.

The mentally healthy person never allows himself to become bogged down with these emotions to such an extent that they dominate both his thinking and feeling. Those who fall into such a trap end up like the man with the perpetual chip on his shoulder, ready to explode, hostile toward everyone and causing every one to be hostile toward him. The mentally healthy person manages to cope successfully with life's problems and challenges even though it may take considerable effort. Much of this involves the need to deal with the challenges and difficulties of each stage of life—what pioneering psychoanalyst Erik Erikson has termed the developmental and psychological tasks of each phase.

These tasks must be dealt with successfully at each age before we can move on to the next one: the adolescent, for example, must free himself of his ties to his parents and mature both physically and emotionally before he can hope for a happy successful adulthood. The tasks that face those in their sixties and beyond are perhaps the most difficult of all; the losses grow and increase, become more pronounced—losses both physical and psychological, of loved ones and of jobs—while the rewards become fewer.

For the emotionally disturbed person, these tasks become exaggerated, the unfortunate events that happen to us all seem much bigger and more threatening than they really are. The problems that can be mastered or brought under control by the mentally healthy person become overpowering to the emotionally disturbed—he feels helpless and defeated. As the NIMH experts explain: "He loses his grip . . . Life has him on the run." The pleasures that should go with living pale into insignificance beside the unhappiness and deprivation he experiences. His life becomes grim and forbidding.

HOW COMMON ARE EMOTIONAL PROBLEMS?

Mental health problems are truly everybody's business today and are not limited to those over sixty-five, although in these later years such problems may take special forms. The most commonly used figure for the number of Americans needing mental health care is 10 percent, but even that figure now seems to be obsolete. The President's

Commission on Mental Health reported on September 1, 1977: "There is new evidence that this figure may be closer to fifteen percent of the population."

We have already seen the psychosocial pressures on the elderly: the attitudes of our society epitomized by mandatory retirement; its concepts of ageism and "senility;" the well-known economic problems of the elderly. One would expect a higher rate of mental illness among older Americans, but it is a tribute to their hardiness that NIA has found it to be no greater than among the rest of the citizens of this country.

NIA reports that some 15 percent of those sixty-five years and older "are in need of treatment or intervention to maintain their mental health." But also note this further comment of vital importance (confirming Dr. Braceland's views): "Those elderly thus afflicted are responsive to treatment if or when appropriate treatment is developed and provided." Unless both doctors and public understand this point, however, understand that the older person has emotional problems that are primarily connected with his or her *humanity* and not with age, and that these are amenable to treatment and cure—then that older person may be condemned with a quick diagnosis of "senility" and sent off to an untreated and hopeless institutionalized half-life.

Final proof lies in two classic community mental health studies conducted in mid-Manhattan and in Stirling County, Nova Scotia. They indicate no significant increase in mental illness with age. And to further hammer home the nail, Dr. Ewald W. Busse, Duke University professor of psychiatry and a pioneer in geropsychiatry, estimates that only between 2 and 3 percent of our elderly are in institutions as the result of psychiatric or emotional illnesses!

The rapid growth of our general mental health problem is highlighted in many ways. Dr. John H. Knowles, President of The Rockefeller Foundation and former General Director of Massachusetts General Hospital, says that "mental illness is *the* major health problem of the United States—and we may see an increase in that while we see a decrease in somatic diseases such as heart attacks, strokes, cancer and so on."

The proof of Dr. Knowles' belief is there: both the mid-Manhattan and Stirling County studies found that 60 percent, nearly two-thirds, of the general population suffered with psychosomatic problems. And a team headed by Dr. John J. Schwab, professor of psychiatry at the University of Louisville, reported to the sixth World Congress of Psychiatry in Honolulu in September 1977 that "psychosomatic illness is reaching epidemic proportions in the Western world." His team conducted a countywide Florida health study of the frequency and distribution of eleven psychosomatic disorders among nearly 1700 adults between the ages of seventeen and ninety-two and found that roughly 40 percent reported weight problems or headaches; some 20 to 35 percent had a variety of stomach and intestinal difficulties (indigestion, stomach aches, nervous stomach, constipation); 15 percent had had diarrhea or hypertension; and about 2 to 3 percent told of peptic ulcer, asthma, or colitis. Slightly more than half of the total population had at least one of these psychosomatic problems "regularly" while 17.3

percent had two or more—almost exactly corresponding to the Manhattan and Stirling County figures.

But what are the red flags of such problems?

THE WARNING SIGNALS OF MENTAL HEALTH PROBLEMS

ANXIETY: fear and anxiety are similar yet different. If you saw a lion running down the street at you, you would have a normal fear reaction—your heart would start racing, your breath would come faster, a cold sweat would break out, your muscles would tense, and all body systems would rapidly prepare themselves for the classic "fight or flight" reaction. In short, fear is a protective measure that Nature developed for your safety. However, if all these same physiologic reactions occurred to you when there was no lion or other real threat, if you had fear without real cause, a sense of impending doom without reason, that state would be considered anxiety. This ever-present anxiety indicates an underlying emotional problem, calls for a medical consultation at the very least, and perhaps specialized help such as psychotherapy.

PSYCHOSOMATIC SYMPTOMS OR DISORDERS: as we have already seen, these are the physical ailments, complaints, or symptoms that have no physical or organic (somatic) basis. They may range from tension headaches to butterflies in the stomach, diarrhea to backaches, an eye twitch to intestinal cramps, and include pain of any sort. In all these cases, there is no physical basis for the ailment at all, but nevertheless these victims do suffer, do feel pain. The physician must be consulted to determine whether there is in fact any disease present or whether the complaints are psychosomatic. Specialized help may be needed here too.

DEPRESSION: this is the most common emotional illness today and involves so many serious, complex issues, particularly for the older person, that it has been deliberately set aside here to be considered in detail in the next chapter.

ABRUPT CHANGES IN MOOD AND BEHAVIOR: others may be aware of these alterations before the individual realizes it himself. Such changes are not meant to include deliberate alterations made by a person to improve himself, such as deciding to make his clothing more modern or to be fussier about how he or she dresses; but it does mean such things as becoming depressed when good things happen (winning the sweepstakes, say, or getting a desired new and better job), throwing money around promiscuously when the individual has always been frugal, or drinking heavily when he's always been a teetotaller. Professional help may be needed here too.

PERFECTIONISM: this may well involve unrealistic and superidealistic demands on oneself or one's employees or family, demands that no one could possibly meet. If the individual cannot discuss and recognize his or her overdemanding attitude and make adequate compromises with reality, a healthy and satisfying emotional life becomes impossible and professional help is needed.

HYPOCHONDRIASIS: this is particularly common after the age of sixty and among women—an overconcern with one's physical or emotional health, with the belief that part of one's body is either diseased or not functioning as properly as it should be. It is so significant among older people that we will discuss it at greater length a little later on in this chapter. However, where this persists professional help should be sought.

There are other warning signals as well, but these are

the most important for the elderly. What produces these disturbances?

THE CAUSE OF EMOTIONAL DIFFICULTIES

A host of professions and disciplines have been engaged for a great many years in the search for the basic sources of mental and emotional illnesses, yet the causes are so complex, so intertwined and interrelated that they have proven to be immensely difficult to sort out. Many observers feel there is no one cause but a whole legion of factors operating together and separately to produce each individual's unique situation.

We have already heard Dr. Braceland's point that the behavior ordinarily thought of as "senility" is often emotional and not physical, and he adds, "The saying that one is as old as he thinks and feels is not simply a flippant remark." We have also seen how many people whose brains have undergone considerable physical changes exhibit no functional effect. Further, Dr. Busse, one of the major figures in gerontology and geropsychiatry, concludes from the famous Duke Study of the aging that "dementia in late life is a social socio-psycho-somatic disorder," and notes that "the loss of mental ability in late life is not usually the result of solely a pathologic brain change," but, as he puts it: "The loss of mental ability (what one does) and capacity (what is possible) is influenced by changes within the brain, the health status of the entire body, behavioral patterns, and socio-economic determinants." With so many complex factors it is not surprising that the clinical course of such patients is one of periodic flareups, unpredictable ups and downs, recoveries and recurrences.

The individual's environment, however, can be critical. As the NIMH experts put it: "The person . . . needs to feel respected, important in the scheme of things, and valued at home, on the job, and at play." One need only look at our society's attitude and treatment of the over-sixty-five person to realize that America is virtually doing everything possible to destroy his mental health. It attacks him at every single point enumerated: at his self-respect and importance, at his place in the home, at his job, at his leisure activities. The amazing thing is that older people are so flexible, tough, and self-reliant that they can survive such destructive environmental factors and keep on functioning. The tragedy is that these attitudes and manners of treatment provide the background for high levels of depression and suicide—one-quarter of all suicides are older than sixty-five, even though the age group makes up only a little more than 10 percent of our society—but we will probe this in detail in our next chapter.

Now let's look at the chief emotional problems that the older person must face—and the way to deal with them.

LOSS, ADAPTATION AND NEW GROWTH

On the surface, one's later life—despite the pretty title of the "Golden Years"—tends to look like years of pure loss: loss of youth, physical strength and vigor, hair and sometimes teeth as well, hearing and perhaps some sight, of societal respect, of job, of relations and friends. But what is commonly forgotten or simply ignored is that the later years should be a time of growth and new development as well.

As Erikson pointed out, old age too has its tasks—and

all too often in our youth-oriented society we think of growth as stopping somewhere in early middle age. Not long ago I interviewed a nationally known young surgeon (he was just forty) who told me in all seriousness that no one ever accomplished anything after his mid-forties!

The reasons for this attitude are fairly clear. In youth, and even in early middle age, the gains (growing up, raising a family, reaching the top in one's business) so far outweigh the losses (losing parental protection, seeing one's children grow up and leave, and the like) that the balance is all in favor of gain. After sixty-five, however, the losses begin to mount up—but there *are* gains, and it is essential for the aging person to keep them in mind. His developmental task in this last stage of life is to continue and fulfill his development, to integrate and consolidate all he or she has learned and achieved in a lifetime, to clarify his wisdom and judgement and find ways to put them all to use.

This has always been recognized; statesmanship and sagacity have always been regarded as a particular possession of the elders of a tribe or community or nation. The very expression "elder statesman" makes this clear and anyone can tick off names, from Ben Franklin to Bernard Baruch to Charles de Gaulle to Golda Meir.

If the person who moves into this last stage of life can still grow and develop, he can look forward to the next day, for it will always carry the excitement of discovery that it had when he was young and each day promised some new experience. As a ninety-year-old patient once told me: "There are still a lot of things whose working out I would like to see." And another, in her mid-eighties, looked forward eagerly to each election because she could work for the party of her choice making phone calls and doing volunteer office work. I have seen it too in a great many other people I've interviewed in their seventies and eighties, people who are all still growing, still tackling questions whose answers hang out there waiting to be discovered by some daring and adventurous mind, ever-young in its capacity to grow and change.

Without this adaptive capacity, the rapid pace of progress, particularly in this Space Age world we live in, can leave the older person feeling threatened, confused, alone. The frequent result is anxiety.

ANXIETY IN THE LATER YEARS

We've already described the symptoms of anxiety—the sensation of impending doom, the physical manifestations of the "fight or flight" reflex—muscle tension, rapid heartbeat, cold sweat. Just the awareness of the oncoming of age is enough to precipitate these feelings, and often the simple security of physical and psychological circumstances that will not suddenly be changed or snatched away will help to relieve these anxieties. Tranquilizers and sedatives can relieve these feelings, too, but they are given much too often and if prescribed or taken on a regular basis for long periods can produce the very thing these same prescribing physicians would label "senility"—loss of memory, confusion, even disorientation or delirium. Unfortunately, this reliance on pills is so widespread that in 1975 antianxiety drugs were one of the most frequently prescribed medications in America, their sales alone totaling a quarter of a billion dollars. Treatment here should be what it is for other, younger people: psychotherapy.

SLEEP DISTURBANCES

This is another common problem of aging. Sleep patterns change throughout life but the reasonably healthy over-sixty-five person needs no more than seven and a half to eight and a half hours of sleep a night, even though many older people physically spend more than this time in bed. However, the time it takes to fall asleep does increase with age so that many older people take at least twenty minutes to doze off where it only took some eight to twelve minutes when they were younger. In addition, older people are more likely to wake during the night and then stay awake longer. Also, adult women sleep differently from men, spending more time in bed and sleeping more but waking up less often than men.

This matter of sleep arouses a great deal of concern among Americans in general (just listen to people at work talking of how well or how poorly they slept the night before), and the elderly who have new patterns to contend with are very disturbed; doctors can testify to the complaints and the pleas for help. Dr. Busse feels strongly about the way Americans behave toward sleep: "It's important for older people to understand that sleep patterns do change, differences do occur—sleep happens to be an important change because there are too many TV advertisements which suggest that people are supposed to have some perfect type of sleep, are supposed to go to sleep promptly and sleep uninterruptedly—as if there were some ideal. Too many people are likely to start taking medications unnecessarily when they are just behaving like all normal people and really don't require *any* medication at all."

We will discuss this American problem of pill-popping further in Chapter 7.

HYPOCHONDRIASIS AND THE GOLDEN YEARS

Dr. Busse was one of the first to investigate hypochondriasis in elderly people and defines it, as we mentioned earlier, as "an anxious preoccupation with one's own body or a portion of it that the person believes is diseased or functioning improperly." Hypochondriasis is a disorder with many meanings; it sometimes serves, for instance, as a means of communication with family or medical professionals—most of us have at one time or another played sick to escape facing up to some difficulty. This "sick role" is especially utilized by older people for a variety of purposes: to center psychic interest on oneself, to punish oneself for anger toward someone close, even to deal with anxiety.

Dr. Busse: "We do know that a substantial number of elderly people—probably about a third of any group of so-called reasonably normal people getting along in the community—do end up with excessive bodily concern. This does not necessarily mean that they go to the physician but it is quite likely they will buy over-the-counter drugs or be overly concerned with diet and so on."

As for how this takes place and why, he explains: "In many of these people it seems to be an interaction between losses within their social environment and finding opportunities to maintain their self-esteem. All people need to feel they have a role in society—that someone really feels they are making a contribution not only to themselves but to others as well. Some elderly people simply go through a period of life when these opportunities are not readily available to maintain their self-esteem. And if, in addition, during a period when they are being deprived of their usual ways of maintaining self-esteem, they are also put into a situation where they are likely to be criticized, then we find they are very likely to become hypochondriacal."

In essence, the hypochondriacal person is saying, "See, I'm sick, don't criticize me." This becomes a way of explaining to themselves and to others why they don't do things or aren't performing as well as people want or expect them to—why, for example, they're not performing their tasks at work or at home.

But then there is a very real problem that strikes the older person . . .

GRIEF AND LONELINESS

As one gets older, losses due to death increase—relatives, friends, even one's spouse. The grief that follows the death of someone close is a normal process and follows a virtually predictable pattern—and knowing that pattern may help relieve the fear it sometimes inspires.

The first days or even the first week following the loss of a loved one is a period that Nature kindly cloaks in a protective veil of numbness, a period of shock and disbelief through which nothing penetrates. When the shock wears off after a week or so, however, the real pain starts, the acute grief filled with memories and thoughts of the lost one; there is crying and sighing and sleep disturbances, too much eating or almost none at all, no interest in anything. It all peaks some two weeks to a month after the death, but things don't really begin to ease until some three months have passed. The acute stage may last six months or so, after which things finally begin to come together as the pain softens, acute distress turns to sadness, remembrance includes some pleasant memories, and interests begin to reappear. By the end of approximately a year, normal life has usually resumed with all its outside interests and involvements.

Latest studies indicate, however, that mourning (particularly for a spouse) may well go on for one, two or even three years—longer for a widow than for a widower. Like any sickness or injury, grief takes time to heal and requires a long, slow, painful recovery process. Eventually, healing does take place, though, and the emotionally healthy person acquires new interests, new relationships, and eventually a new life.

For the elderly, particularly, a loss always brings up the specter of loneliness, which is not a matter of simply being alone: one can be "lonely in a crowd" and even those in nursing homes or homes for the aged often complain of loneliness. Loneliness is the absence of truly meaningful relations with other human beings—and life's satisfactions can be found in the quantity and quality of such ties. Loneliness or social isolation seems especially felt by those who have lost a husband or wife while those who have always been single complain much less often. It is loss and not simply physical isolation that is the key. The best remedy is a determined effort to make new friends—and perhaps to find a new mate.

ATTAINING MENTAL HEALTH IN THE LATER YEARS

NIMH experts have some simple effective suggestions for helping people maintain a state of mental health or achieve one. There is no magic to these steps; they are simply grounded in observed facts, things we all really know deep down. The person who is tense, anxious or angry will tend to stir up similar feelings in those with whom he is in close contact, and their defensive reactions to this behavior will make things more difficult in turn for the person who is already uptight. Start yelling at someone and he'll get mad too! The behaviors that the experts suggest are simply means for reducing the frictions and tensions of life, for making it run a little easier, a little more smoothly—for making it possible to deal more effectively with life's problems.

THE "EASY DOES IT" APPROACH: this is simply intended to gain cooperation from those with whom one deals. If you avoid overreacting to the problem, you can be in control of the situation and make whatever compromises are needed so as not to antagonize those who don't fully agree. This also implies an ability to see the real goal. If you know what you are really trying to accomplish on a larger scale, then you can give on the minor unimportant issues while achieving your chief aims with a minimum of friction.

HELPING OTHERS: this is not Pollyanna-thinking but a real, hard fact—the moody, disturbed person unable to take effective action can break out of such a situation by trying to help someone else. Alcoholics Anonymous utilizes this principle and has found it very effective: when members are in danger of drinking they seek to help someone else with the same problem and in this way help themselves over the crisis.

TRYING TO ANALYZE AND HANDLE YOUR ANGER: understanding why you are angry often helps to control this potentially destructive reaction. Frustration—trying to open a stuck drawer or being harassed by a superior on the job where anger must be controlled, for instance—may lead to a flareup at an innocent bystander (your wife or husband, a shopkeeper). Knowing and admitting the real reason for anger often helps, but another good way is to blow off steam with a sensible trustworthy friend or with a clergyman, doctor or even a professional counselor.

DON'T BROOD: doing something positive or useful in a situation is more valuable than simply stewing about it. Doing something else—a change of pace—focuses energies on something useful and constructive and is a simple way of getting away from it all, of avoiding simply racing one's motor.

PROCEEDING ONE STEP AT A TIME: it's the trapped feeling that is so deadly. Once you start moving toward a solution—however slowly—a feeling of self-worth results from being able to handle the situation. We should all learn to channel our tensions and angers toward worthwhile and reachable goals. Learning to function this way can be a slow process, particularly in the beginning, but you can gain a surprising degree of control over how smoothly your world runs. Ultimately, the most important factor is yourself.

The truth of this statement can be seen from a story Catherine O'Donoghue, director of the Aging Program at the Menninger Foundation, tells young psychiatrists in training. A woman in her mid-nineties was taking correspondence courses while working toward a master's degree; she got back one test with an F grade and was furious because she always did B or better. Protesting the grade, she learned she'd missed answering some questions and was offered an oral examination. She took it and got her B. Unknowingly, she used virtually all the principles of mental health described above, and showed how effective they could be.

One further tip: Dr. Daniel T. Peak, Medical Director of the Continued Treatment Unit at John Umstead Hospital in Butner, N.C. sees a way to secure mental and emotional health in the later years by developing "the ability to arrange or rearrange our lives so that we are able to live within our capacities and within our environmental setting, and in the process achieve a sense of well-being." In other words, learning how to be happy with what you have. For this, he notes, a person must have five things: "flexibility, an awareness of one's limitations, a knowledge of one's options, a store of resources, and the ability to achieve a sense of well-being."

HELP FOR EMOTIONAL PROBLEMS

Once the prejudices and distortions of ageism are set aside, the emotional problems of the older person are seen to be no different than those of the younger one. Even though each age group is unique, and has its particular needs, once it is recognized that the old dog *can* learn new tricks, psychotherapy can intervene in the emotional problems of the older person just as successfully as with younger people.

As Dr. Braceland points out: "The management of the emotional problems of non-organic aged persons [those who do not have chronic brain syndrome, OBS] is neither as difficult nor as futile as is generally believed." Psychiatry has changed its opinion considerably over the years. All those who work with the elderly agree that as patients they are very receptive to help, with results that are satisfying to patient and therapist alike.

All the traditional individual and group psychotherapeutic techniques are applicable, but there is one unique form of therapy that Dr. Butler finds of enormous value to the older person in particular. It's called "life review therapy," and in it the individual conducts virtually a verbal autobiography by way of memories and even memorabilia—the family album, say, or scrapbooks—to bring out past events of important emotional significance that can lead to increased self-understanding. The goal of this therapy is to resolve and relieve guilt feelings and inner conflicts, to reconcile family members and settle old problems, even to pass on the knowledge and values of the older person to those who are to follow.

Health conditions alone demand more flexibility in therapy for the elderly. Dr. Butler urges that therapists be flexible about the use of the telephone for psychotherapy when patients can not come in personally because of physical limitations or disabilities. He tells of one elderly man who suffered from a heart condition and so would call when he could not travel to the office; he had his therapeutic session by phone (although he did manage to keep nine out of ten appointments).

Group therapy has also been widely used for older people and serves some special functions. It offers, for example, the socialization that older people so often lack. The skills gained in relating to others in a group can then be turned to advantage in gaining membership to groups outside the therapeutic situation. Moreover, the oldest person in the group is often listened to by the others, giving him improved self-esteem as well as showing the others that they all share in the same problems and that these can be solved.

So today the way to mental health and to the resolution of one's emotional problems are available to people *regardless* of age. Truly here is an opportunity to add life to one's years.

There are two other major psychological problems that often must be confronted, however, and the next chapter deals with those.

CHAPTER 6

Conquering Depression and Suicide, the Great Enemies of Age

DEPRESSION AND suicide are twin destroyers of the elderly—and two of man's most ancient enemies. Depression is as frequent among the mental ailments as the common cold is among the physical—and some even say that depression is second in overall occurrence only to the common cold. Fifteen percent of all Americans, some thirty-two million of us, will suffer each year with this potentially deadly disorder—perhaps even as many as a third of us, depending on your definition of "depression."

The deadliness of depression comes chiefly from the suicides with which it is so closely involved. NIMH experts point out that of the suicides reported each year in the United States, "more than eighty percent are believed to be precipitated by depressive illness"—and there are an estimated 50,000 to 75,000 suicides each year in our country. Both depression and suicide have a very special meaning for the elderly: they are much more common among our older citizens, are, in fact, a very frequent problem; and although over-sixty-five Americans make up only slightly more than 10 percent of us, they provide a startlingly and disproportionately high 25 percent of all our suicides.

In this chapter we will look at the background of depression and suicide: who they strike, what depression is, how to recognize it, how it can be treated, and how understanding depression is already helping to put an end to "senility." We will also look at suicide—who is most likely to try this drastic step and what danger signals to watch out for.

DEPRESSION AND SUICIDE: THEIR HISTORY AND THE VICTIMS THEY STRIKE

Depression—once known as melancholy or melancholia—seems to go as far back as man himself. It can be found described in ancient Egyptian medical papyri, parts of which date back 6,000 years, and in the Old Testament, which so often tells simply of human problems. King Saul suffered from depression—an evil spirit, the Bible reports—and David provided music therapy with his harp to relieve it. *The Book of Job* itself can be used as virtually a clinical textbook of depression with its psychiatrically accurate description of depression, the physical manifestations, and even the roles of the therapist or comforter and the sufferer. Hippocrates, too, described depression under the term melancholia.

The strange thing about this mental ailment is that it seems to damage the genius of its victims very little; the roll of those who have suffered from it reads like a Who's Who, from Nathaniel Hawthorne, Edgar Allan Poe, and Dostoyevski to Winston Churchill and Abraham Lincoln. Josh Logan, director and co-author of *Mr. Roberts* and *South Pacific*, among other hits, was tormented by it, but performed brilliantly; U.S. Senator Thomas F. Eagleton of Missouri has a history of depression and electroshock that cost him the vice-presidential nomination in 1972, but it never kept him from functioning effectively and creatively as a member of our Senate. And James V. Forrestal readied our Navy for World War II, directed its vast wartime expansion and development, and became our first Secretary of Defense while suffering from it; unfortunately he later succumbed to depressive illness and took his own life.

Suicide, too, is a very old phenomenon—human beings seem to have been bent on carrying out their own self-destruction since virtually their first appearance on this planet. There has evidently never been a society without suicide: it was known in India some 5- or 6,000 years ago, there are four recorded instances in the Old Testament, including Saul and Samson; and it was an ancient tradition in Greece and Rome. The incidence of suicide in modern times is well known; no chapter on the history of suicide is complete without some mention of the suicides of such as Vincent Van Gogh, Virginia Woolf, Ernest Hemingway, and Sylvia Plath, as well as the attempts—or at least threateningly deep depressions—of Washington, Lincoln, Napoleon, and Bismarck.

Cultural attitudes toward suicide have varied markedly

over the ages. Most societies have condemned it. On what is now the Aegean coast of Turkey, a curious epidemic struck the greatest Greek city of the Near East, Miletus. In about the fourth century B.C., the young women of that community were stricken by a rash of suicides; despite all the attempts of their families to prevent it, they persisted in hanging themselves. From this behavior was born the first official suicide-prevention measures. The magistrates of Miletus decreed that the bodies of those who hanged themselves would be carried through the marketplace to their burial—and the threat of such shame even after death finally brought this wave of self-destruction to its end. Unfortunately we seem to have no effective societal measures available today.

The ancient Greek and Roman societies viewed suicide with some ambivalence. On the one hand, it was considered an "honorable" way out for a warrior or statesman in an impossible position; on the other hand, it resulted in a very material financial loss to those owners whose slaves indulged in it. In medieval times the Christian Church considered suicide a form of murder inspired by the devil, and acted accordingly: the bodies of suicides were mistreated in various ingenious and degrading ways, as in England, where they were dragged naked through the streets, hung upside down, and even impaled on a stake.

Thus society has usually declared suicide taboo and acted in a variety of ways to enforce that taboo. Not even the recognition that suicide arises from troubled and desperate human minds has served to remove that stigma. Even today society makes the families of the self-destructive feel almost like criminals. Religious attitudes are condemnatory, life insurance companies punish them by refusing payment of benefits unless the policy has been in effect a certain period (commonly at least a year or more), and cultural attitudes are still so strong that in most cases the family tries to deny the act and almost invariably seeks to conceal it publicly by claiming that it was an accident—an overdose of drugs taken by mistake, for example, or someone falling out of a window while confused by sleep. Physicians, too, try to avoid labeling a death as suicide, not only when they treat the family but even when acting as official medical examiners.

Depression and suicide are most democratic in their natures—they strike the high and the low, the creative artist and the businessman, the scientist and the statesman alike. Nor is there any hint of sexist attitude; both men and women are stricken . . . although there is a marked sex difference in suicides, as we shall see.

But first let us take a look at the problem of depression.

DEPRESSION AND "SENILITY"

H had abruptly or gradually become apathetic and yet restless; he was fatigued and neither ate well nor slept properly, had lost weight and suffered with insomnia. He'd also become somewhat confused, inefficient of memory, and unable to concentrate, his attention continually drifting away from whatever was being discussed.

If H were thirty-eight or forty, even fifty, years of age, his doctor would be concerned and insist on carrying out a thorough examination and careful evaluation of the problem. Suspecting a depressive illness, the physician would likely suggest a psychiatric consultation if he felt the situation was beyond his capacity to handle properly, but in any case he would be optimistic, hopeful, and encouraging with patient and family alike, insisting on the excellence of the outlook and urging a positive, active medical approach and treatment. He would be right, too, for the hope for depressive illness today *is* excellent and the chances are at least eight or nine out of ten that H would be back functioning as he always had within a month or two.

But if H were sixty-five or seventy or more, most physicians would become only minimally involved, would take a pessimistic view of the future, offer a gloomy forecast, and make little attempt to active treatment. The doctor would carry out little in the way of tests or examination or evaluation ("no sense wasting money unnecessarily"). The diagnosis would simply be "senility"—and that would be the end of that. In point of fact, however, depression is much more common in the elderly than in the young—yet the outlook is just as hopeful, given the same degree and quality of care, interest, and knowledgeable treatment. Regardless of his age, H has the same chance of recovery as anyone, unless the mythical diagnosis of "senility" causes him to be sent to a mental institution or nursing home where he is likely to get neither adequate medical nor psychiatric care.

Recently Dr. Karl A. Menninger recalled a typical ward in a local hospital more than thirty years ago. It was a ward in the Topeka State Hospital devoted to the elderly with all the symptoms of "senile dementia." Of eighty-eight such patients, fifty-one had been bedridden for an average of a decade, about twenty even needing spoon-feeding—in short, a group of incontinent and hopeless shells.

An eager young physician came in with a team of bright, joyful young nurses, social workers, and residents. The gloomy ward was converted into a bright hospital-home with pretty curtains, birds, plants, and TV. The patients were involved in parties and their relatives actively invited into the situation. The patients themselves began to participate and made changes to physically improve the actual construction of the facility.

Three weeks after all this began, one patient was discharged. By the end of the year twelve more had gone home to their families: six to live by themselves; four to pleasant nursing homes; four were working and self-supporting. Five had died and only nine of the original eighty-eight were still bed patients! Here is actual proof of how "senility" can be brought to a dramatic end—simply by putting an end to depression!

DEPRESSION: WHAT IT IS AND HOW IT SHOWS ITSELF

Depression is not an easy condition to understand: doctors disagree about the classifications, diagnosis is difficult and often uncertain, its presence is often missed because it is hidden. For example, it may only show itself as a headache about which the sufferer will typically report, "I've had a headache every single day of my life"—now we know that chronic pain is often "a depressive equivalent" (so-called "masked depression"), a symptom that signals that the real underlying problem is depressive illness. In fact, depression often shows itself not in what a person says or feels (not in "being blue" or "down in the mouth"), but in the symptoms he possesses (difficulty with sleep, chronic pain, constipation, fatigue, and a host of others). Confused? That's not surprising, because doctors usually are, too, and it often takes a really good psychiatrist to recognize this strange disorder.

Depression is an emotional state, an "affect," as psychiatrists put it, a feeling-tone of sadness that can vary from the mildest of blues—downhearted, in the dumps, mildly discouraged—to utter black despair in which there is no longer any glimmer of light or hope. Winston Churchill called it his "black dog" and Ishmael in *Moby Dick* talked of "this November in my soul."

It's the most common of psychiatric complaints, but it's one that follows no classic or precise pattern and has no usual or specific outcome. It may be mild, moderate or severe; acute or chronic; fleeting or lasting—may vary from a mere passing shadow to the severely crippling illness that ultimately ends in suicide. It may even turn itself completely around and show itself as depression at one stage and as elation or excitement at another (psychiatrists often speak of this as bipolar or manic-depressive illness as compared to unipolar depression).

Another common distinction is between reactive and endogenous depression. Reactive depression is primarily a response to some outside event such as the death of someone close, the loss of one's job, or a serious rejection or misfortune such as the author whose major book is condemned by the reviewers. These are commonly self-limiting reactions and with time (getting over the loss) or improvement of the situation (a new job, better reviews) usually lifts. Endogenous depression, however, arises from deeply rooted sources within the victim, from his unconscious mind and often from unconscious guilt; it is also suspected by many psychiatrists to be associated with somatic or organic causes—with actual biological factors.

Depression can proceed along a continuum from mild to moderate to severe, with virtually no marked or sharp distinctions. The milder forms of depression are characterized by varying degrees of unhappiness and pessimism, feelings of inadequacy and loss of interest in the world; conversation may be difficult and the ability to think affected; there may be feelings of unreality and a variety of physical complaints or depressive equivalents, as well as bewilderment; difficulty with the performance of ordinarily simple mental activities and even an inability to make decisions. One patient I knew would walk into a store to buy a loaf of bread and, confronted by a variety of brands, find himself unable to decide on which to purchase and, finally, leave without any.

As one moves into the more severe forms, the victims show marked behavioral changes, a constant tension, and an impenetrable absorption with a few gloomy subjects; delusions, self-accusations, and feelings of guilt, sin, and unworthiness are common; any replies to questions are monosyllabic and halting; the facial expression is one of hopelessness and dejection—the mouth sagging, the forehead furrowed, the eyes directed downward. The preoccupation with depressive meditations may be so great that memory, concentration, and even attention may be impaired (compare this with the conventional picture of "senility"), and, finally and most seriously, thoughts of suicide become frequent.

Frequently, too, a variety of physical symptoms accompany depression, such as loss of appetite, weight loss, insomnia (particularly complaints of awakening early), constipation (the entire intestinal tract becomes sluggish), lack of energy and chronic tiredness, decreased sex drive, and a variety of pains (headaches, menstrual cramps, stomach complaints; chest, back, joint, muscle, and other pains). These often confuse the physician, who may treat only the symptoms and so accomplish nothing.

Despite the long history of the disorder, however, the cause of depression is still not fully clear—and there are two schools of thought, although these may yet prove to be only one. Many believe that emotional or psychological problems are at the root of depression, while a newer school looks to the neurotransmitters, those chemicals that permit neuronal messages to pass across synapses, as the cause. Ultimately, the source may prove to be a combination of the two—changes in the environment stirring up biochemical changes or the other way around.

But depression in those over sixty-five is somewhat special . . .

DEPRESSION IN THE ELDERLY PERSON

There is some difference between the depressions of younger and older people. For one thing, recurrent spells of depression (which may actually last only a few minutes, or a few days at most) are common in the elderly. Older people themselves, as studied by Dr. Busse and others, are aware they have more frequent and more troublesome periods of depression during which they feel disheartened, troubled, even disgusted with what they felt and saw as their own uselessness.

The cause of depression also seems to differ somewhat. Guilt, for example, generally plays a relatively unimportant role; but the losses of later life may bring the elderly person to the point where he feels he has lost everything and that nothing is left—which would certainly make any one feel depressed. Loneliness, too, is a problem and can itself lead to depression.

As Dr. Busse of Duke University reports: "Not only do elderly people develop depressions that require medical intervention more frequently, but they also report more periods of depression—down periods—during a normal day or normal week and most people working in this area of geriatrics agree that these do increase. I think we always have to look for the interaction between the biological changes and the adverse or perhaps destructive or negative environment in which a person may be struggling to function."

There is another factor as well: biochemical changes in the neurotransmitters. Dr. Busse continued: "A number of investigators hold that a chemical called monoamine oxidase (MAO) increases in the aging brain. Since MAO is an apparent element in depression, there would appear to be some truth in the belief that the elderly person is physiologically predisposed to depression. It would appear then that we have an interaction between the changes in the body with the passage of time which may make elderly people more vulnerable to certain adverse social conditions." And the ageism of our heavily youth-oriented society makes it likely that the elderly will be exposed to both societal and self-criticism, which can lead to *further* loss of self-esteem—which can lead to further depression.

What can be done about all this?

THE TREATMENT OF DEPRESSION

Dr. Leslie Libow sums up the treatment of depression in the older person this way: "Depression is very treatable once it's properly diagnosed—it is treated best with simple medications; at times with psychotherapy either individual or group; at times with a combination of chemicals and psychotherapy; and occasionally, in severe depression of such severity that the individual needs to be taken care of twenty-four hours in the day either at home or in the hospital, where he is profoundly depressed and cannot function, with electro-convulsive therapy [ECT—electroshock], but this should be used only in advanced cases of depression."

Virtually all the experts today agree with this therapeutic pattern, and Dr. Busse adds that the profoundly depressed older person should be hospitalized because of the very high risk of suicide, and because the depth of the depression is best determined and treatment most effectively given in a hospital. Furthermore there is the risk that the victim may recover spontaneously and then return to the very situation that created the problem in the first place.

Psychotherapy is most commonly used in conjunction with other forms of therapy since it is less likely to be sufficient by itself. Extremely depressed patients, for example, are very limited in their ability to engage in the dialogue necessary for psychotherapy and, moreover, its beneficial effects take time, if they can be achieved at all, and meanwhile there is both the severe suffering and the great danger of suicide to reckon with.

Since 1957 a growing number of drugs have proven to be very useful in fighting depression. These include MAO inhibitors (for example, Nardil and Marplan), but the ones usually tried first are the so-called tricyclic compounds, a group of powerful mood-elevating compounds of which Tofranil and Elavil are common examples. These are powerful drugs and are available only on prescription, and should only be prescribed by doctors thoroughly familiar with their properties, uses, and actions in the elderly person. In older patients these drugs can have troublesome side effects, particularly on the central nervous system and the cardiovascular, so they must be used cautiously and monitored very closely by the doctor.

One drug that has received a lot of publicity is a naturally occurring chemical element called lithium, which in 1949 was found to calm manic patients. "Mania" is a sort of mirror image of depression, the other half of manic-depressive illness, and its symptoms are enormous elation, optimism, and euphoria—"I feel like a million bucks," "I can lick the world." In this stage, the sufferer feels all-powerful and may be hyperactive, speak rapidly, and even have delusions of vast capabilities to achieve unlimited and unrealistic ends. In 1970, lithium was approved for use as a prescription drug because clinical research had shown it to be able to relieve not only manic symptoms but also manic-depressive episodes; studies since then have even indicated that it may benefit the unipolar problems (repeated episodes of depression) as well. However, there is still some question as to whether the use of tricyclic antidepressants and lithium for extended periods may cause serious side effects, and NIMH has only recently begun a long-term clinical study to clarify the situation.

Finally, when all of these measures fail, ECT must be considered. The mythology, fears and misunderstandings that have gathered about this treatment are so great that the therapy warrants some detailed exploration.

ELECTROCONVULSIVE ("SHOCK") THERAPY: THE FACTS AND THE FICTION

By whatever name you call it—electroshock, shock, electroconvulsive therapy—ECT has always aroused man's ancient fears of helplessness, with its fantasies of grim-visaged medical technicians assaulting one's brain. As a result, attacks have been made on it, and recently its image was even more aggravated by the movie *One Flew Over the Cuckoo's Nest,* in which Jack Nicholson was given a science-fiction kind of ECT as a punishment. The truth of the matter is that electroshock treatments are an ancient technique: the Egyptians were putting drawings of the Nile's electric catfish in their murals nearly 5,000 years ago; and some 2500 years ago Plato and Aristotle knew that the electric torpedo fish could make a human limb go numb. Nero's most famous surgeon, Pedanius Dioscorides, advised using the electricity from this fish for headaches by applying the whole fish to the head.

In 1934 a Viennese physician, Manfred Sakel, discovered that large doses of insulin caused convulsions, confusion and then a deep sleep. It was an extremely dangerous procedure, but was quickly hailed as an effective treatment for schizophrenia—for a little while. Its effectiveness was later called into question by most medical authorities, and it is used very rarely today. Only three years later, however, in 1937, two Italian neuropsychiatrists, Ugo Cerletti and Lucio Bini, discovered ECT. At first nobody recognized it as a specific for depression and applied it indiscriminately in a way that makes one shudder today; some patients were given as many as fifty or one hundred treatments during a few months' time. Fortunately, the damage was not great—one young patient who had received more than one hundred treatments, for instance, later attended a university and earned a doctorate.

ECT has come a long way since that time, however; its use has matured and been developed and refined. Today the usual course of therapy runs somewhere between four and ten treatments over a period of two to three weeks, and a recent study revealed one leading psychiatric hospital using ECT on only 7.5 percent of its patients. Both here and in England studies have proven ECT the most effective treatment for depression—it can clear the depression in one or two weeks where the antidepressant drugs take roughly twice as long to be effective—and an NIMH study found it at least moderately beneficial in 93 percent of its depressed patients.

Properly used, ECT today is both simple and safe. The patient is prepared before breakfast with an injection of a barbiturate and a muscle relaxant and when he is unconscious, two electrodes are placed on his forehead, either one on each temple or both on the same side. The actual shock (less than a hundredth of a volt) lasts a tiny fraction of a second and the only movement of the patient is some slight shaking of the toes—the great body-shaking convulsions of the past were the result of less sophisticated techniques. The person awakens several minutes later and can then have breakfast—and if desired he can even walk home with a companion an hour or two later, although this is usually not the case. If he's sick enough to need ECT, he's sick enough to stay in the hospital rather than at home.

While the patient will experience some confusion when he first wakes after the ECT, this clears after a few minutes and any temporary memory loss will soon remedy itself. Again, this is usually only a matter of a few minutes after the person regains consciousness, although some loss has been demonstrated up to twenty-four hours later and some people complain of even longer bouts. This is an unclear area because, although there have been patients who have reported memory difficulties months or even years later, it is not always certain how good their memories were before ECT—those with serious depressions who have never had ECT also show memory problems. Most psychiatrists feel that the side effects of ECT are sufficiently minimal—or entirely absent—so that they do not represent any drawback.

How exactly does ECT work? Just as doctors have yet to puzzle out the exact mechanism of depression itself, in the same way the precise workings of ECT (as with aspirin) remain a mystery. Many experts believe, however, that the electricity affects the neurotransmitters in the brain. While one course of treatments is usually all that is ever needed, some patients do have to continue taking antidepressant drugs after ECT.

And then there is suicide.

SUICIDE IN THE ELDERLY

The cause of suicide still lies buried deep in the human soul and mind—a mystery like so many other things about us. Although it has long fascinated man, it remains an enigma, an act whose meaning, whether a cry for help or an attempt to escape suffering, seems to vary with the individual. When it takes the life of someone past the age of sixty-five, however, the act is doubly ironic for it negates the suicide's own long struggle of nearly three-quarters of a century or more to survive—a task successful despite all the threats and difficulties and odds, only to be wiped out in a meaningless gesture.

Despite man's long acquaintance with suicide and his attempts to deal with it by societal taboos and laws, it is still with us and by far its greatest toll is among the aged. The suicide figures for both the young and the elderly are startling, and perhaps if we were more aware of their drastic number we would do more about them. This is even truer for attempted suicide, where only the tip of the iceberg shows. As Dr. Herbert C. Modlin, director of preventive psychiatry at the Menninger Foundation, points out: "Traditionally, suicide has been avoided in polite civilized conversations, reflecting a strong mystical taboo. Little wonder that our statistics concerning the incidence of suicide are incomplete and unreliable." A British study revealed that in 1960 and 1961 there were ten times as many attempted suicides as successful ones; a Los Angeles survey found the same proportion; a Swiss study indicated a ratio of *fifteen* to one—and these figures include only those incidents in which a physician was actually called in.

Official records indicate some 24,000 suicides a year, but the actual numbers are thought to be two or three times as high, making a rough total of some 50,000 to 75,000 deaths. Using the studies above, we can then put the numbers of those who *attempt* suicide at some half million to a full million annually. In short, one or two Americans attempt to commit suicide every minute—and roughly 150 to 200 succeed in their tries every day. Put this against the fact that those over sixty-five make up one-quarter of all suicides in America and the numbers are truly alarming. A federal estimate of the suicide rate of those fifty-five to eighty-four—made in 1972—shows it to be almost double the average for all ages put together, and the rate increases with each decade of life as we age, peaking among men in their eighties.

There are marked sex differences in suicide—three out of four successful suicides are carried out by men while the figure is the same for *unsuccessful* suicides among women: twice as many women as men attempt suicide and fail. A number of reasons have been suggested for this difference. Stress and the pressures of the world seem to be involved—during business recessions male suicide rates jump an average of nearly 10 percent a year while those of women barely move (less than 3 percent). In addition, American men tend to keep their problems to themselves, and are expected not to cry or seek help but to be self-reliant and brave. This blocks them from seeking help and leads them to a stage of lonely desperation more often than women, who can cry or lean on husbands or friends for support and even use the suicide attempt as a cry for help. Moreover, men commonly use weapons such as guns for suicide, which leaves little chance for medical help, while women turn to poisons, from whose effects medical rescue is still possible. Then, too, men are more likely to drink, and this, as we shall see later, is important.

A final factor influencing suicide rates are those stresses and pressures peculiar to a particular society. Dr. Ari Kiev, a Cornell University professor of psychiatry formerly in charge of their Social Psychiatry Program (chiefly concerned with suicide), notes that in the Orient women kill themselves more often than men and he concludes this is "a cultural and not a biological sex difference—it suggests certain stress factors pertaining to the role of men in our society." And Dr. William R. Cunnick, Jr., Deputy Chief Medical Director of the Metropolitan Life Insurance Company, calls attention to its figures showing sharply upward trends in suicides among younger and middle-aged women during the last two decades. As he points out, this was a period during which many women took jobs, with all the accompanying stresses, and became the heads of single-parent families. He concludes: "The achievement of 'women's liberation' has not been without its costs."

HOW CAN SUICIDE BE PREVENTED?

Suicide is one problem that cannot be treated—it can only be prevented—and at this particular time the only hope for prevention seems to be a matter of pinpointing the potential victim and getting help to him or her in time. There were high hopes for suicide prevention centers in the 1960s, but unfortunately they were soon dashed because it was found that the telephone therapy—the so-called "hotlines"—that most suicide prevention centers utilized simply did not reduce the level of suicides. Ultimately, the NIMH Center for Studies of Suicide Prevention was closed down in the early 1970s.

However, suicides can be prevented and there is help available—but instead of "hotlines" it is the family, friends, and doctors who must form the first line of defense. The key to prevention lies in Dr. Modlin's observation that "Homicide is frequently impulsive; suicides almost never." Thus there is almost always warning beforehand.

THE RED FLAGS OF SUICIDE

"The patient at maximum risk for suicide is an older, white, divorced, unemployed male who lives alone and is in poor health," Dr. Modlin points out. He is especially susceptible to depression, and depression is one of the single most important criteria of suicide potential. Hopelessness, loneliness, helplessness—all of these are strong factors commonly noted in suicides, and should be watched closely.

Even the time of year can be a warning. A Duke University study has recently been confirmed at the University of Minnesota: T.S. Eliot was right when he wrote that "April is the cruellest month"; March would seem to be the peak month for depression and April for suicides. Psychiatrists have a simple explanation for this: the depressed person sees the light and new life, the growth and happiness of spring, and it contrasts so sharply with his own dead feelings and unhappiness that he can finally no longer tolerate it.

Increasing age in itself can be a warning that one should be on the alert for other signals. With age and the destructive attitudes of our society, the elderly person can lose his self-esteem and anything that decreases this—a disappointment, a loss, an emotional blow, an illness, the need for surgery—can possibly lead to suicide. Moreover, the older person is increasingly aware of his own weaknesses and, as he ages, the helpless feeling grows that there is no road back from any of his losses, that he is losing control over the world around him.

Any talk of suicide must be taken seriously, particularly when the individual has any of the danger signals mentioned above. Remarks such as "I'm tired of it all," "I can't take it any more," "I've just had it," "Life isn't worth living," and the like should not be ignored. Actions, however, may speak louder than words and many suicides—especially among the elderly—don't talk about it at all. Instead they may show it. They may, for example, have the physical symptoms of depression. Abruptly or radically changed behavior patterns are particular danger signals—the suicidal person may suddenly turn contemplative and remote, lose interest in eating and sex, talk little, in short begin to withdraw from the world about him; or he may suddenly start to give away prized possessions, discuss insurance policies, rewrite a will, secure a weapon or a large supply of sleeping pills.

The very opposite may also signal danger of suicide, however. As Dr. Kiev explains: "Someone in the midst of a depression may suddenly dramatically improve and even become a little euphorically elated—this frequently happens when someone's made a decision—'Enough of this depression, I'm going to kill myself and get it over with.' Then they begin to feel a lightening of the pressure on them."

While virtually every one of us has thought at some time or other, "I wish I wasn't here," or something like it, such thoughts usually occur under particularly bad pressure when everything has been going wrong for weeks, and occupy only a passing few moments before disappearing. This is not really a danger signal. When the thought becomes frequent and recurrent, however, that *is* a warning. The myth that those who talk about suicide don't commit it is sheer nonsense—any talk about suicide must be taken seriously and help sought from experts; we'll talk about who to turn to in the next section.

Another dangerous myth is the belief that those who attempt suicide and fail are just "putting on a show" and don't really mean it. The fact of the matter is that once a person has attempted suicide he has broken a major protective psychological barrier, he's in the big leagues now and is at serious risk. Clinical studies have shown that anywhere from a quarter to nearly two-thirds of those who succeed in committing suicide have tried to do so before, and the suicide rate among previous attempters is sixty-four times higher than that in the population as a whole.

Another major factor in suicides is drinking. Dr. Kiev's studies pointed out that perhaps a third of the patients studied had been drinking excessively. Contrary to popular belief, alcohol actually makes a person more, not less, depressed, so the depressed individual is in even greater danger. Moreover, if a person has had a bad day and then starts to drink, feelings and reactions that he can normally block out of his consciousness come to the surface, and the reaction can be severe. Drinking affects one's judgement as well, causing one to do something one might not ordinarily do. Dr. Kiev warns: "When you're depressed you shouldn't drink!"

Finally, watch out for the person who is accustomed to acting impulsively. If something disturbs him (fired from his job, a fight with his wife or the like) he can then walk out and step in front of a car or turn a gun on himself.

THE CARE AND PREVENTION OF SUICIDE

Dr. Kiev explains that, "Nobody really wants to kill himself—he just doesn't want to go on feeling the way he does." It is difficult for the ordinary person to comprehend fully the terrible blackness, the utter hopeless despair of the person in a severe depression, the fervent desire to end it in whatever way possible. So the first step in prevention is to get any depressed person to seek or accept medical or psychiatric help in bringing the depression to an early end. It's important too that the physicians the person sees be competent, for there is a sad lack in general understanding by doctors about this whole matter of suicide.

A recent study of practicing California physicians by Drs. Don A. Rockwell and William O'Brien of the University of California revealed that nine of ten physicians recognized the inadequacy of their knowledge of suicide. To make matters worse for the elderly, 86 percent of these doctors were ignorant of the fact that older persons are the most likely age group to commit suicide.

While the family practitioner may be capable of dealing

with depression, it is probably best, when confronting suicide, to seek someone with specialized knowledge in the field—most likely either a psychiatrist or clinical psychologist. The situation can be discussed with a knowledgeable family doctor, however, as long as he is aware of his own limitations and can suggest the proper suicide expert or clinic; if this referral is not forthcoming or obtainable, a call to the nearest medical school or university-based teaching hospital will bring information on either a local suicide clinic or expert if a private practitioner is desired. You are dealing with human life here and the best is none too good in the way of help.

But what the concerned friend or relative or mate can do is mostly on the negative side—what not to do. Certainly, always take any suicide threat seriously and seek professional help promptly and work closely with the expert. But Dr. Calvin J. Frederick, former assistant chief of the NIMH Center for Studies of Suicide Prevention, warns of the danger of anything even remotely resembling a challenge to the suicidal person: telling him "You're not the type," or "You don't mean it." It's like waving a red flag; indicating disbelief in the suicidal threat may be just the challenge he needs to go ahead with it. The magazine of the American Medical Association reports one instance: threatening to kill himself a suicide climbed to the family roof, then moved listlessly, uncertainly to the edge. One of the onlookers in the street below shouted up in a sneering voice, "Go ahead and jump"—and the suicide promptly did just that.

Another common error—the superpositive, overcheerful "Come on, snap out of this" attitude—as Dr. Kiev warns, "increases the load on the individual and weighs against the desire to live, the individual's basic force for life." And to tell him, "Come on—you'll feel better," or "You've got everything to live for, you're terrific," or "You don't have to feel this way," only creates still further problems, as the Cornell psychiatrist explains: "This only deepens their guilt and self-blame, makes them feel frustrated and angry and that nobody understands how they feel—and they may develop a pressing need to escape such crippling distress, for just before the actual suicide attempt the tension turns minutes into hours and days into unending nights. They can't imagine this state is really brief and self-limited."

Obviously with such complex mechanisms in operation—and a human life at stake—expert professional help is utterly essential. With such help, however, the outlook can always be positive, for today there are a multitude of approaches available both for depression and for suicide.

In the next chapter, we will look at some closely related problems.

CHAPTER 7

Drugs, Diet and Alcohol

THE MAN was checked out thoroughly before he entered the large western medical center for surgery and, as was customary in his type of surgery, an antibiotic, gentamicin (a close relation of streptomycin), was given to prevent infection. Suddenly the patient became disoriented and confused, even began to have hallucinations. Doctors made a diagnosis of acute organic brain syndrome, OBS, and had the man been over sixty or sixty-five instead of well under it, the cause might very well have been put down as "senility." Instead the difficulty was traced to the antibiotic, the drug was discontinued and the OBS promptly cleared up. There have been a half-dozen instances now in which this antibiotic was the source of readily reversible OBS, and each instance stands as a cautionary tale of the unpredictable effects of drugs and medications of all sorts on man. This problem is particularly acute in the elderly due to their changed physiology, but it is not always recognized—sometimes to tragic results.

Medications are not the only causes of reversible OBS in the elderly. Another very common problem is that of malnutrition, brought on by loneliness, neglect or poverty. Lonely elderly people, of whom there are some twenty million in America, may well lose all interest in preparing meals; burdened with grief (particularly over the loss of a spouse) or with the emotional discomfort of being alone, they end up merely eating toast and tea, and perhaps some milk. The result, as NIA Director Butler points out, is: "We often find ourselves admitting such a person to a hospital with what gets referred to very easily as 'senility,' but is simply inadequate food supply to the brain." The brain needs food just to function properly and clearly, without confusion.

Here again we have the myth of "senility"—this time as the result of improper diets or nutrition, or the effect of drugs. In this chapter we will look at the problems of both drugs and diet, as well as a newly discovered problem—the elderly alcoholic.

THE PILL-POPPING PROBLEM

One of our greatest dilemmas is the way our society turns to pill-popping, abetted and even encouraged by the medical profession. Studies completed in the early and mid-1970s reveal the startling extent of our involvement.

Unfortunately the act of writing a prescription is an effective technique for ending a visit satisfactorily for most patients as well as for doctors: the patient feels he or she has had something "done" for him or her, the doctor doesn't have to spend too much time on the patient and doesn't have to deal with his or her emotional problems. Also, if a physician is uncertain of the problem and not too secure in his own competence or knowledge, he feels safer in prescribing an antibiotic—he's covered should the trouble prove to be an infection—and patients overvalue antibiotics because of their long-standing reputation as "miracle drugs."

Dr. Paul D. Stolley, Johns Hopkins professor of epidemiology, has pointed out, for example, that nearly two-thirds of all common colds treated with medication by doctors are really being *mis*treated. The common cold is a virus infection and 60 percent of the prescriptions given for it are antibiotics that have no effect on viruses. Similarly, in a study done by Dr. James A. Visconti, director of Ohio State University Hospital's Drug Information Center, in a 500-bed community hospital it was found that one-third of the more than 1,000 patients admitted during a one-month period had been given antibacterial drugs—and more than 87 percent of these had been prescribed irrationally.

In one mid-Atlantic community Dr. Stolley found that the two types of drugs most often prescribed were antibiotics and psychoactive or mood-altering drugs (sedatives, tranquilizers and the like). The total number of prescriptions dispensed in 1970 was more than two billion, with some 350 million of these going for psychoactive drugs. In that year alone, the drug industry turned out five billion doses of tranquilizers, five billion of barbiturates, and 3 billion of amphetamines! Two-thirds of the physicians in a Harvard Medical School community survey by Professor David C. Lewis agreed that too many prescriptions were being given out—and more than half the druggists surveyed agreed that the public themselves were buying too many mood-altering OTC (over the counter without the need for a prescription) drugs.

Besides the danger of becoming habituated to drugs, there is the perhaps greater and certainly increasing danger of adverse drug reactions—from rashes to diarrhea to serious kidney or blood complications—or of drug interactions that can themselves lead to adverse reactions or at least negate any positive effect. A study at the University of Florida Teaching Hospital in Gainesville by Drs. Ronald B. Stewart and Leighton E. Cluff revealed that their seventy-five subjects took a total of 245 prescription (Rx) drugs, as well as a wide array of OTC medications. One patient was found to have taken fourteen drugs in a thirty-day period, another thirteen, two others eleven each. Hospital charts rarely showed fewer than ten to fifteen drugs for a patient and one patient's chart actually listed forty-three drugs. Furthermore, a computerized study of the prescriptions given some 42,000 Californians showed that 84 percent of the patients were being given prescriptions that presented serious problems of drug interactions.

The public too is at fault here. The Social Security Administration did a study comparing the amounts of Rx and OTC drugs taken, and in terms of dollars they found that during 1969 Americans spent $2.6 billion for OTC drugs and $4 billion for prescriptions—both figures virtually double what they had been just a decade before. While no one can tell how many OTC items are sold in any one year, it is possible to reach an estimate from data published in medical, hospital and druggist magazines of some *1,866 million* prescriptions filled in the United States that year. With the usually higher cost for Rx drugs we can only guess at how many more OTC items were bought.

This whole problem of an overmedicated America is compounded where the elderly are concerned because of their increased health difficulties. Dr. Busse has shown in a series of important studies that more than three out of four people over the age of sixty-five have one or more chronic illnesses (illnesses lasting longer than three months) as compared to two out of three people between forty-five and sixty-five, and less than one out of two in their early adulthood. Also, the severity of these illnesses increases with age and, after reaching seventy-five, some 24 percent are unable to carry on their major activities because of these chronic disorders, as compared to 10 percent of those between sixty-five and seventy-four years of age.

The use of drugs and the risks they represent have special meaning for older people, for with their many chronic illness problems it is not surprising to find that although those over sixty-five represent a little more than 10 percent of our population, they purchase a full one-fourth of all prescription drugs. In 1974 this group alone spent an estimated $2.3 billion on such medications. Add to this all the OTC drugs they purchase and you have the makings of major adverse or paradoxical drug reaction problems.

The overall picture is clear. According to Dr. Robert E. Vestal, professor of medicine at the University of

Washington, the average older person spends almost one hundred dollars a year for prescriptions and OTC drugs, and averages over thirteen prescriptions annually. And he is much more susceptible to adverse drug reactions: in 700 Johns Hopkins Hospital patients, 25 percent of those over eighty had adverse reactions compared to only 12 percent in the forty-one to fifty age bracket. Furthermore, a recent University of Florida study revealed that 3 percent of over 6,000 hospital admissions occurred because of adverse drug reactions—and of those who suffered these reactions nearly half (41 percent) were over the age of sixty. Similar percentages have been reported in Great Britain as well.

The dangers of drug overuse and abuse are everywhere and drug use in America is mind-boggling at times. In 1971, for example, Americans spent $600 million on OTC painkillers (analgesics) alone, and this included $105 million for aspirin, $387 million for aspirin combined with other drugs, and more than $63 million on products for arthritic and rheumatic pains. Yet for that year prescriptions for analgesics ran *third* in frequency behind psychoactive drugs and antibiotics. Add it all together and one has such vast purchases of analgesic drugs that it is virtually impossible to conceive of a nation so pain-wracked that such huge amounts of relief are truly needed.

Even with such a seemingly safe drug as aspirin a whole host of adverse reactions and interactions is possible. Aspirin can even kill; adults have been known to die from as few as three tablets. It can set off severe asthmatic attacks or bleeding in those who are allergic to the drug; it can cause bleeding in those who are taking blood thinners (after heart attacks, for example) or those with peptic ulcers; it can cause problems for those taking gout medication or prescription drugs for diabetes or those who have hemophilia. Yet with all this, it can be so safe that arthritics have taken a dozen or fifteen or more aspirin a day for ten or twenty years and more. Here indeed is a drug that shows it all—safety when properly used, but danger and even deadliness when used by the wrong people or combined with the wrong drugs. It is a good example, in short, of the importance of a simple precaution: the older person should always check with his doctor before taking any new drug—or even before taking a drink of alcohol if he is on regular medication.

DOCTORS, THE TAKING OF DRUGS, AND THE OLDER PERSON

We all change as we get older, and one of those changes is that our metabolism, the sum total of all the chemical reactions that take place in the human body, slows down. This includes the operations of the liver and the kidneys, the chief organs that first alter or break down, then eliminate, drugs. Kidney action, for example, is said to be reduced by a third between the time a person reaches his twentieth birthday and when he makes it to his eightieth. Body water content is reduced, as is plasma (the liquid part of the blood), and body muscle is replaced chiefly by fat and fibrous tissue, in which drugs often accumulate. With less fluid, too, there is a greater concentration of any drug, alcohol for example, and the increased fat raises the amount of drug retained by the body when a medicine is taken. As a result, the half-life of medications—the time it actually takes for 50 percent of a drug to be eliminated from the body—is increased. Vanderbilt University investigators have found, for instance, that Valium, probably the most frequently prescribed drug today, lasts four or five times longer in older people. As a result, Valium can easily accumulate to an excessive degree, with serious mental side effects if prescribed by a doctor for a man of seventy in the same dosages as for a man of thirty. In addition, Dr. Busse suggests that the loss of brain cells may make the older brain more sensitive to certain drugs.

Unfortunately it happens all too often that neither the older person nor his physician is aware of the problem—and the result is "senility" (actually acute OBS) induced by the wrong drugs or the wrong dosages or the wrong instructions for taking them. The number of medications capable of causing drug reactions in elderly persons is vast: steroids such as cortisone used for arthritis may produce acute or chronic OBS in the older person; barbiturates ordinarily thought of as sedatives and used as sleep-aids may paradoxically cause excitation; some tranquilizers may lead to depression or a dangerous drowsiness, causing accidents; water pills (diuretics) may cause dehydration and result in mental confusion.

NIA Director Butler is particularly concerned about this problem: he tells, for instance, of how a certain type of tranquilizer, the phenothiazines, when given to the elderly for a long time can "create a terrifying horrible condition called tardive dyskinesia: the victim has no control over his mouth area and his tongue reaches out as though it were trying to catch a fly."

As he points out: "Obviously, drugs have a very important place in health care, but we do tend to overuse them, to misuse them, and to have insufficient knowledge about their relationship to age. Our doctors learn from textbooks which do not even have 'age' in their indexes. . . . [they] may be quite unaware of the possible drug-drug adverse interactions and of the age-drug interactions that can and do occur." There are at least one million Americans of all ages who suffer adverse drug reactions every year, and some 30,000 die from them, so it is essential that the older person be aware of such reactions and of what they are for each drug he takes, and doubly careful in his choice of a knowledgeable doctor. Our next chapter will tell how to do this.

HOW THE ELDERLY CAN PROTECT THEMSELVES AGAINST MISUSE OR OVERUSE OF DRUGS

In the older person, Dr. Butler warns, "even the tranquilizers and antidepressants have to be used with extraordinary care because you get much more of a wallop with the same dose than you would when you're younger. The older person should be very questioning about the use of drugs—should ask the doctor if a more modest dose could have the same effect—and I don't think more than one drug should be introduced at the same time in the older person, if possible. In threatening situations, such as extreme heart failure, you have to give a number of different agents simultaneously, but in the more general situations, I like to introduce them slowly, one after another on different days and see just what the effects are, monitoring the patient very carefully."

If the older person is taking medications for a variety of conditions simultaneously, especially if he is being treated by several different specialists or clinics at the same time, it is essential that he inform his regular doctor of just what drugs he is taking. This is why having a general or family doctor is so important—he can orchestrate the total medical picture, making sure that the drugs for the patient's arthritis don't interact with what he may be taking for congestive heart failure, for instance. This, too, is why self-medication can be such a problem—the older person should always check with his doctor before even taking aspirin.

Then there is alcohol. Alcohol, too, is a drug, and there is a wide range of medications that react badly when even a single drink is added, and some of these reactions have even been fatal. No one taking medication should ever take an alcoholic drink without asking his doctor beforehand.

THE NEW ALCOHOLIC PROBLEM IN THE ELDERLY

Traditionally, alcoholism has been considered a disease of younger people, its incidence peaking between the ages of thirty-five and fifty. Either things are changing, however, or we are only now becoming aware that it is an older person's problem as well. For example, the *Detroit Free Press* reported in 1977 that ever since the United Auto Workers won new retirement privileges four years earlier their Memorial Hospital's alcoholism treatment unit had seen a dramatic rise in older patients. Typical was their story of a former city employee who had been drinking for forty years with no apparent difficulties until retirement—only nine months later he was under treatment for alcoholism.

Confirming stories abound. A major house-to-house survey in Manhattan's Washington Heights section in 1965 revealed the peak incidence of alcoholism to be in those aged forty-five to fifty-four, with twenty-three per thousand afflicted—but effectively tied with them were those sixty-five to seventy-four years old with an incidence of twenty-two per thousand, or 2.2 percent. Surveys have shown that elderly widowers have the highest rate of alcoholism of all the subgroups in our population—105 per thousand. And older *women* have been drinking more heavily as well, as indicated in an Alcoholics Anonymous study noted in a report on alcohol and health by the National Institute on Alcohol Abuse and Alcoholism (NIAAA).

A survey of hotlines—telephone referral services—is reported to have found about a third of all calls for help on alcoholism coming from people over the age of fifty-five. Sun City, Arizona, an affluent retirement community of less than 40,000, not only has three Alcoholics Anonymous chapters but also a special therapy group for recovered alcoholics. The staff of St. Luke's Hospital in Phoenix, Arizona, nationally known for its alcohol and drug rehabilitation programs, has found its case load of elderly patients so heavy that it has actually started a special therapeutic program just for them. And of nearly 600 patients over the age of sixty admitted consecutively to the San Francisco General Hospital, 28 percent had a serious drinking problem.

There is no question that alcoholism in the aged has reached a critical stage. One expert has calculated that at least one *million* Americans over the age of fifty-five are alcoholics, a figure that should increase as the numbers of elderly and retirees increase, particularly since those over sixty-five today still tend to come out of a background of temperance and relative abstinence.

It is an insidious problem, especially since so many families are unwilling to recognize or admit that a grandfather or grandmother, father or mother, is alcoholic—a difficulty often shared by physicians as well, even when they are able to recognize what is wrong. The roots of the problem lie in the NIAA-quoted now classic study of older alcoholics by Bruce Carruth, "significant isolation, loneliness and other psychological pain." A man or woman drinks to cope or to escape from coping. It is a cry for help from people overwhelmed by loneliness, depression and hopelessness, by grief at the death of someone close, by helplessness at retirement, or even concern over failing health.

It *can* be treated, however. Alcoholics Anonymous can be helpful, of course, and traditional psychiatry. For elderly alcoholics in particular, a program by Dr. Sheldon Zimberg, a professor of psychiatry at New York's Mount Sinai Medical School, combining antidepressant drugs and socialization programs—trips, discussion groups, dressmatches and the like—has met with considerable success. Dr. Zimberg finds alcoholism often is a cry for help from people overwhelmed by loneliness, depression, hopelessness, or grief. With new alcoholics—those who have only lately begun drinking due to the stresses of aging—he has been able to succeed without AA, and even with the chronic alcoholics has been able to obtain long periods of abstinence. It is a spark of hope in what has always been a gloomy picture, and may well make the outlook for elderly alcoholics quite different—

perhaps even better?—than that for younger ones!

Now let us turn to an essential that has all too often been misused.

FOOD, DIETS AND NUTRITION

Food is the very staff of life, one must have it or die, yet too much or too little or the wrong kind can shorten one's life and lead to a multitude of disorders. That Americans are concerned about this fact is clear from the numbers who make best sellers out of any new gimmicky diet book that promises a quick easy way to take off weight, despite its proven effectiveness or lack of it, or even its proven danger.

Man has always been interested in his food, and scientists and doctors have long been concerned with its role in health and disease. We've come a long way; we seem to know how to prevent certain diseases with diet, but that most serious problem, obesity, still affects some 30 to 40 percent of us, cuts life short, and causes disorder after disorder. As Dr. John H. Knowles, President of the Rockefeller Foundation and one of America's great public health experts, explains: "There's plenty of evidence that obesity leads to everything from premature onset of diabetes to strokes and heart attacks, and that excessive fat in the diet and obesity are associated with certain forms of cancer." In fact, the outlook for the obese person is so poor that a common hospital locker room joke is: the best way to treat a very obese person is to give him to a doctor you particularly dislike. Many physicians now regard obesity as *the* major American Health problem.

Yet the exact incidence of obesity is not really clear—

nor, actually, is its precise definition. In general, the adult who weighs twenty *pounds* or more over what tables say he should is regarded as obese. This number includes 30 percent of American men and 40 percent of American women. Others use a yardstick of twenty *percent* or more above the ideal weight figures, while a third method has the doctor pinch or lift a fold of skin over the triceps of the arm, and then measure the fold with a special pair of calipers. He then compares this figure to a special set of standard tables to reveal the actual amount of body fat and determines whether the patient is obese or just heavily muscled. A ten-state federal survey using this more precise test found that among Americans aged sixty-five to seventy-four, some 15 percent of the men were overweight and more than a third of the women.

Whatever the test, do obesity and diet really influence heart disease? While there is still some argument, the experts seem increasingly to agree: yes. For instance, in 1976 Dr. Kaare Norum of Norway's University of Oslo sent out a questionnaire to 214 medical scientists engaged in research into coronary heart disease in twenty-two countries. Nine out of ten answered, and virtually all (more than 99 percent) agreed there was a tie-in between diet and heart disease, and the same number also saw a connection between the amount of cholesterol in the blood and heart attacks (coronary heart disease). About 92 percent believed a moderate dietary change to reduce calories and saturated and total fat should be recommended. Their opinions were supported by a November 1977 University of Chicago research report that affirmed that hardening of the arteries—accumulation of fat deposits in the inner linings of the blood vessels, also known as atherosclerosis—in rhesus monkeys could be stopped and even reversed by a restrictive low-fat, low-cholesterol diet.

This pattern of reducing elevated blood lipids such as cholesterol in the blood by modern dietary techniques led Dr. James A. Schoenberger, professor of preventive medicine at Chicago's Rush-Presbyterian-St. Luke's Medical Center, to say recently: "For the first time a downward trend in coronary artery disease in the United States has been reported and changing patterns in the national diet have contributed."

There is still some lingering controversy over this whole area of dietary manipulation, however, and before any person tries to alter his own diet he should consult his doctor, simply because there may be some very personal health problem that precludes or makes the particular change unwise or unnecessary. Moreover, changes in diet must be done knowledgeably so that no important nutritional elements are lost—and must be done with an awareness of any medication being taken, for even diet can interact with drugs and special diets may be needed when certain drugs are used or certain diseases present. Diet is much too complicated and essential to health for the untrained person to fool with.

Apart from this specific problem of cholesterol, what other nutritional guidelines should the older person follow? Here is what the experts say. First, Dr. Robert E. Shank, professor of medicine at Washington University (St. Louis): "The nutritional requirements of older persons are not importantly different from those of younger individuals. The most important difference is in reduced requirement for calories, which reflects the reduction in basal metabolism and decreased physical activity. . . . Although requirements for the essential nutrients are not significantly changed for older persons, food habits and preferences as well as social, economic and environmental characteristics do change. Diets may be quite different from those consumed by the same persons in earlier life. Important factors affecting diets are: decrease in taste sensations, return to childhood food preferences, edentulousness [loss of teeth], social isolation, loneliness, and decreased income.

And Dr. Jean Mayer, former Harvard professor of nutrition and now President of Tufts University, points out: "The quality requirements for minerals, vitamins and protein are not less for elderly people, but with less total food intake the density of nutrients has to be greater, which unfortunately is not always the case. Put everything together and what you arrive at is not a special recipe for nutrition in old age—you won't be immortal if you feed yourself well—but you can make your old age more comfortable by practising the elementary rules of nutritional hygiene. . . . The quality of the diet must be preserved: people must be educated to the value of the primary foods—fruits, vegetables, meat, fish, eggs, milk and whole grain cereals in particular. Older people must have sufficient calcium, iron, protein and vitamins.

"Overweight prematurely ages people and accelerates the medical consequences of aging. A diet high in fats—particularly in eggs with their high cholesterol, in fatty meats, in cream, in hydrogenated vegetable fats—tends to elevate people's cholesterol and cause premature hardening of the arteries. Another very common condition in both middle and older age is high blood pressure; a diet high in salt seems to predispose people to this and we as a nation tend to salt an awful lot of things."

And Dr. John Knowles adds: "Finally, reduce the use of refined carbohydrates or sugars as compared with those in natural fruits with their high fiber content, for refined ones can conceivably lead to the premature onset of diabetes."

Beware of fad diets. Often their recommendations have no solid basis in fact, or they can even prove dangerous, as was the case with the recent liquid protein diet. After more than two dozen deaths were reported in those taking liquid protein, the federal Food and Drug Administration, in the person of FDA Commissioner Donald Kennedy, felt compelled to issue a public warning that said, among other things, "On the basis of the information we have to date, we have every reason to believe that the liquid protein diet was at least a contributing factor or a cause of the deaths."

Again, before even considering any of these diets, consult your doctor, even if only by telephone. Even the safest of diets may be extremely dangerous to a particular individual because of his or her own medical problems—and picking the wrong diet may well be taking one's life into one's own hands.

Which leads us to the next chapter—how to pick the right doctor.

CHAPTER 8

The Fight for Medical and Emotional Help: How to Find the Right Doctor

WE'VE ALREADY met Dr. Butler's engineer whose healthy stubbornness alone kept him from being "put away" in a nursing home or mental hospital as "senile" when all he had was a viral infection. Editor Robin Marantz Henig tells, in the medical magazine *The New Physician*, of three patients who weren't that lucky. Two were women in their mid-seventies and the third a man in his mid-eighties. One of the women had always been alert and independent but, like the engineer, became confused, disoriented and terrified; she too was diagnosed as having chronic OBS (the usual "senility"), but her misfortune was that her viral infection was never recognized. She was sent to a nursing home. The other woman was troubled by a general out-of-sorts feeling and seemed confused when she appeared for her regular medical checkup; her doctor sent her home with an Rx for a tranquilizer and told her it was to be expected at her age. Her real problem was appendicitis, however. In older people, as we've seen, the classic symptoms of diseases are often missing, so she showed no pain or abdominal tenderness or temperature. Similarly, the man in his mid-eighties was told, together with his family, that his disorientation was normal at his age; but the truth was that he had suffered a heart attack, and, again, he had had none of the classic symptoms, no chest pains or breath shortness.

This sort of problem is widespread in America today. For a variety of reasons—current medical training, expertise, attitudes, even the age of most physicians—it is a real struggle for the older person to obtain proper medical and emotional care. Let's look at how the older person or his family can choose the right professional man for the increasing health needs of later life, how the doctor's qualifications can be checked, and why it is sometimes difficult to find him.

HOW AND WHY DOCTORS GET THAT WAY

Underlying it all is America's built-in ageism, societal attitudes in which medical students and doctors alike get trapped. Their personal prejudices often get started when, as medical students, they meet their first older "patient" in the shape of the cadaver supplied for dissection. Few of our medical schools show any interest in their students' reactions to these dissections—their nausea and vomiting, confusion and nightmares. Left to their own devices, the young people attempt to cope with these disturbing reactions through "gallows" humor, and, as NIA Director Butler points out: "Youth-oriented Peter Panism, or callous and cruel epithets such as "crock," "turkey," "toad," and the one I just heard—"dirtball"—become synonymous with the older person." A study of University of California medical students has shown that these attitudes toward the elderly in fact get worse during the course of their medical school years.

Such negative images of the aged are not surprising since the only elderly these young doctors-in-training commonly see are the sick, the deteriorating and the degenerating—and then the unconscious images stick throughout their professional careers. Unlike their frequent opportunities to meet healthy infants and children during their training, students never get to see what healthy, vigorous, attractive older people can be like—there isn't a single American medical school that routinely rotates its students through the active community senior citizen centers.

Moreover, medical students traditionally model themselves on the professors with whom they come in contact during their training and this is what attracts them into particular specialties. Whereas England has fully ten professorships of geriatric medicine, little Sweden two and even minuscule Holland one, it was not until 1977 that the United States finally established such a professorship, at Cornell University Medical College—and the school hasn't even been able to find a properly trained expert to fill the chair. Only popular pressure and steady public demand can improve a situation in which the best recent estimates show that, of some 25,000 American medical school faculty members, less than fifteen have any true expertise in geriatric medicine—and these teach a total of only forty-five elective courses spread among 114 medical schools.

This situation is so bad that the September 27, 1976, issue of *Impact*, an American Medical Association publication, reporting the results of a survey of American practicing physicians, found that 75 percent of the respondents admitted that physicians today need special training in geriatrics. There is a great deal of resistance to medical school courses on geriatrics—but when it comes to the doctor himself or his family he finds he wants the advantages of this specialized help. As Dr. Butler points out, "colleagues who had been indifferent, if not hostile, to the idea of teaching geriatric medicine will call me when illness strikes a mother, father, wife, husband or themselves. Then even they recognize the need for a 'specialty' or 'expertise.' " While the deans complain that there is no room for geriatrics in their crowded medical school curriculum, even though it concerns twenty-three million Americans, they still manage to find room for such new fields as neonatology, the field concerned with disorders of the newborn.

How then can one find the right doctor?

THE RIGHT DOCTOR FOR THE OLDER PERSON

Choosing the right physician presents a double problem for the prospective patient: namely, finding one who not only is knowledgeable, but sympathetic in his emotions and attitudes. The physician himself, once he enters middle age—say, his mid-forties—is likely to be struggling with the approach of what is mistakenly regarded in our society as "old age." He may himself be worried about becoming sixty-five, a time when retirement is mandatory from many active positions at hospitals and medical schools, and may believe the myths of senility and aging that we have discussed throughout this book.

As a result of his personal emotional struggle, his fears and anxieties about his own aging, the physician may look with a jaundiced eye at his patients who are themselves sixty-five or older, for both their age and their growing variety of chronic ailments all remind the doctor of what is ahead for him. If he has not resolved his own feelings about this (and few of us really have, in our ageistic society), he may want to avoid being reminded or having his feelings stirred up—and so he gives his older patients short shrift, brushes off their problems and complaints, avoids looking deeper into their health situation for fear of finding things that will make him more frightened of his own oncoming years. None of this is likely to be on a conscious level, but many physicians, for example, refuse to treat or see patients in nursing homes ("I'm too busy" is the usual excuse), or, if he does, it is most likely to be only a very superficial visit, a quick trip in and out.

The physician is also faced with another emotional problem, wished on him in part by our society that emphasizes success and looks down on failure. The doctor's own training makes him feel his job is to heal and cure, to restore patients to perfect health and youthful vigor—and when he fails to do so he feels inadequate, frustrated, a failure. However, many of the complaints of the older patient—an arthritic joint, say, or a mild congestive heart failure—may be relieved today but are likely to return next month or next year, perhaps even in a worse state; he cannot be restored to total health. This concept of "healing" goes against all that the doctor has ever been taught about what he must accomplish. The result is that he may tend to shy away from his elderly patients, may even avoid them when they're seriously ill.

The first thing, then, is to look at a prospective general or family doctor's age. The very young doctors—those under thirty-five—are likely to be impatient with the older patient, to see him as a "pain in the neck," a "crock," as they did only recently in medical school. Those well into their forties are likely to feel threatened. The optimum age for an older person's physician then is between thirty-five and forty-five, or in the late sixties and beyond: the younger group does not feel threatened and the older ones have had to come to grips with their own aging and are not disturbed by others their own age or older.

The second thing is to find a generalist. It's impossible to diagnose our own medical problems and to decide which specialist we should see, particularly for an older person with many medical problems who needs someone to oversee his total management—to decide which medicine for a heart problem should go with which medicine for arthritis, for instance. The old G.P. has now gone the way of the steam locomotive, however. In fact, today's doctor must know far more than the old G.P. ever dreamed of. Today's generalist is, with rare exceptions, either an internist (a specialist in diagnosis and general medicine) or a family physician (F.P.) specially trained in general medicine. The internist (you will see a diploma on his wall certifying to his specialization in internal medicine) usually has a particular special interest—cardiology, rheumatology, diabetology, or the like—and commonly is more interested in his specialty than in general practice, which he most likely had to do as a way of making a living.

If you get the right internist, he can be excellent, of course, but by and large the F.P. is preferable. The F.P. is a new breed who is interested in all of medicine—a Space Age G.P. if you will—but unfortunately there are still not enough of them to go around; only slightly more than 11,000 F.P.'s exist countrywide, and they are seldom found in the large cities (there are a great many internists in the large cities, however). The F.P.—he, too, will have a diploma certifying him as a specialist, but in family practice—is involved with the family as a whole and so is the most likely doctor to be interested in the older patient.

The ideal physician, of course, is a geriatrician, a doctor who specializes in the care of the older person and so is likely to know all about the drug reactions, physical changes, and medical problems of the elderly. He is the one who will be able to recognize OBS and tell whether it is acute or chronic, who can track down the cause and relieve it if it is acute, who will know where to get help if it is chronic and what to do about it. Tragically, however, even though twenty-three million Americans need this specialist, there are only a handful scattered across the country and the likelihood of finding one is very slight. As a result, the older person must make do with an internist or F.P., but many of these *are* interested in older Americans and can be sought out.

You tell if the doctor is sympathetic toward you. For one thing, if he is patronizing, if he addresses the daughter or son and ignores the older person as if he were a child, or takes the "Isn't he/she cute" attitude—forget it. These attitudes are insulting and degrading to the maturity and intelligence of an older person. Such a doctor should be thanked nicely as the older person puts on his hat and leaves to find an adequate physician. Also avoid the doctor who falls back on the "What do you expect—he's/you're an old man" routine, with its variations—he's not interested or knowledgeable enough to care, or perhaps he has too many emotional problems of his own.

The older person needs a doctor who will treat him with the respect and personal concern needed by all human beings, and society tears down his self-esteem far too much already for him to subject himself to more of the same from this doctor. In addition, the doctor who is prejudiced against the older person can never provide proper medical care nor will he be interested enough to bother finding out about geriatric medicine.

HOW TO LOCATE A DOCTOR FOR THE ELDERLY AND HOW TO TELL WHAT HE KNOWS

Not only are geriatricians scarce but it is impossible to find them the way one would an ordinary specialist. The likelihood of finding courses taught on this specialty at the local medical school or of locating a geriatric clinic at the local hospital or medical center is tragically small—only a tiny handful exist across the country. Thus it requires a roundabout approach to reach someone with special interest or expertise.

One method is to call the department of medicine of the

largest available medical school, university teaching hospital, or medical center, starting with the major institutions first and working down to the local hospitals, then ask for the names of any doctors specially interested in the care and treatment of the elderly. The larger the institution, the greater the likelihood that someone there will be interested in geriatrics. If it is a question of "senility," try the same procedure with the department of psychiatry—geropsychiatrists are interested and do have special expertise in this diagnosis.

If none of these work, the community mental health center should have a section devoted to geriatrics and the people there are likely to know who is particularly interested in geriatrics locally.

If the older person or family already has a regular doctor, the approach is somewhat different. A great deal of medical care could be improved if people learned to handle doctors, to ask the right questions in the right way. People tend to assume, for instance, that just because a person is an M.D. he or she knows all areas of medicine. That simply isn't true. A physician may not volunteer that he doesn't know something, but if the patient were to ask, "Doctor, is geriatrics something you are interested in, a field you keep up with or see a lot of?" he will be much more likely to get an honest "No, I don't." The way is then open to ask for a referral to some physician who is interested in the field.

It may also be quite simple for a relative—a son, daughter, nephew or whatever—to ask his doctor for the name of someone who is particularly interested in or knowledgeable about geriatrics or the care of the older person. In addition, an especially good source of referrals is a floor nurse in the local hospital. Nurses see the doctors all the time and notice the kind of patients they usually handle; they can tell you how a doctor acts with his patients, how effective he is, what kinds of patients he likes to treat, and even how knowledgeable he is in various areas.

A good way to check a doctor is to find out whether he is a recognized specialist in his field (although geriatrics today is still not a recognized specialty or even a subspecialty). This can be done unobtrusively by simply observing the diplomas on the wall, because these will attest to the fact that the doctor has been accredited by the primary certifying board of his particular specialty, for example, the American Board of Family Practice. Being board-certified means that this professional person has fulfilled certain training requirements, both in terms of quality and quantity, and has passed special examinations in his field. It won't tell you if he is better than someone else but it will at least assure you that the particular doctor has a certain basic level of competence and knowledge.

Another test is to find out if the doctor teaches at a medical school—the bigger and better the medical school, the fussier it is about its personnel; and the same is true for the staff of a hospital—the better the hospital, the higher the quality of its staff. In both cases, one can then check on the doctor's rank; the head of a department is likely to be more experienced and better qualified than someone at the very bottom of the list.

Now suppose you've found the right doctor, the elderly person has been given the proper treatment, all the appropriate tests have been given and the smallest detail attended to, and the diagnosis is still chronic OBS. Until recently there was little that could be done for the person, but now, at last, there is exciting new hope, even for those previously labeled "untreatable." The next chapter tells the story.

CHAPTER 9

Treating the Untreatable – The New Way to End Senility

THE WOMAN in her nineties was in a New York State Veterans Home and had been diagnosed as suffering from organic brain syndrome (OBS), Parkinson's Disease, hardening of the arteries, and other problems. She was deaf, couldn't utter a sound that her interviewer could understand, nor answer a single one of seventeen questions specifically designed to test her confusion, disorientation and memory loss. She was included in a trial project to test the effectiveness of a relatively new technique called Reality Orientation (RO), even though there seemed little reason by any conventional wisdom to expect that someone so handicapped by physical and mental illnesses could ever again be able to operate on a functional level.

After only a few weeks of RO, however, this lady began to get around by herself in her wheelchair. She could go from her room to where the RO classes were being held, and started to practice her writing and resumed the reading of books and magazines. After two months she read the entire list of seventeen questions and wrote correct and legible answers to more than half of them. She even began training herself to speak again (there was no speech therapist available), and some three months after this pilot project had begun, upon observing the program director trying to speak to her, she was able to reply with a very clear "I can't hear. I am deaf."

This inspiring story is only one indication of the remarkable healing wind of change that is sweeping across the American medical and mental health scene today. Not long ago such people were being written off as hopeless, condemned to the half-life of the mentally disoriented in state hospitals, homes for the aged, and other such depositories. Now at last light has appeared at the end of the long tunnel of hopelessness. The results of Reality Orientation are so exciting that more and more its principles and methods are being applied in institutions everywhere, from Topeka, Kansas, where it was born, to Glasgow, Scotland, to Tuscaloosa, Alabama, to Montreal, Canada. It is even being taught to families and neighbors to be used at home with their loved ones. No one really knows how many human beings have been reclaimed from the back wards and rooms of institutions and restored once more to contact with the world around them by this technique—or at least have had the downhill drift of their OBS slowed to a halt. For those people, RO is nothing short of a miracle.

THE STORY OF REALITY ORIENTATION (RO)

Reality Orientation began when a compassionate young psychiatrist named James C. Folsom turned his interest to rehabilitation medicine at Topeka's V.A. Hospital, where the Menninger School of Psychiatry got its start. He was troubled by what he saw there: well-cared-for elderly and "senile" patients sitting in air-conditioned comfort in pleasant surroundings with absolutely blank expressions, staring over each other's heads, entirely out of touch with the world. These patients were increasingly unable to care for themselves and incontinent, ever more confused, disoriented and forgetful. Then, in 1958, Dr. Folsom introduced an active pilot program into what had traditionally been a passive kind of care—and was thrilled to see a complete turnaround as many of the patients became active again, began wearing their own clothing, and joining groups where before they had been isolated and uninvolved.

He took this program, which he now called "reality orientation," to a large state hospital in Iowa where he had become clinical director. In the three years preceding his arrival, only 3 percent of the 300 patients over sixty-five in that institution had left the facility "other than by death." He immediately began working with the new elderly arrivals who showed strong signs of confusion and disorientation—and by the end of the first six months of his RO program a full 49 percent had been discharged; by the end of the year the rate had risen to 57 percent.

It was not until the mid-1960s, however, when he was Director of the V.A. Hospital in Tuscaloosa, Alabama, that Dr. Folsom finally saw RO reach its full development and gain such national recognition that a stream of health workers began making the trek to Tuscaloosa to study the program and take it back home with them. Here was a true breakthrough, it was realized—the first proof that it was actually possible to restore the mental functioning of older people with OBS to an earlier and improved level. In short, this psychiatrist had broken through the old prejudices against the aged and the mentally disturbed to show that something could and should be done for those people who had not one but two strikes against them: aged and certifiably "senile" besides.

Now Director of New York's famous ICD Rehabilitation and Research Center, Dr. Folsom sums up his view of the basic problem this way: "I don't believe in 'senility'—what is frequently called 'senility' is actually a dehumanization and depersonalization that is inflicted on people led to believe all their lives that the old get 'senile'—and so they become ready victims when presented with such problems as loss of spouse or job, retirement, lessened ability to work, a stroke or heart attack." In fact, he notes, any sudden stress on the individual, such as surgery, can set off such a problem of "senility."

He illustrates how this can happen: a man in his eighties is in an auto accident and undergoes hip surgery, finally awakening from anesthesia to find himself in a strange room. No one calls him by his name or identifies himself (his sons say "Dad," his wife, "Dear"; the nurse enters to turn him over without a word and gives him an injection). There is no calendar or clock visible, the blinds are drawn and he can't tell night from day. He calls his present wife by his dead wife's name and one son by another's name, but no one corrects him. He's given sedatives to make him sleep and he awakens again in a different room. Thoroughly confused by now, he sees someone standing over him with a pillow and thinks he's going to be smothered; he struggles and is tied down and given a stronger sedative. Because of his age he's diagnosed as "senile." He's also likely to be sedated more heavily as he grows more confused and disoriented.

But now someone familiar with RO steps in. Everyone—doctors, nurses, aides, even porters—addresses him by his name, identifying themselves and explaining what they are going to do ("I'm Mrs. Jones, your nurse, and I'll give you an injection to . . ."). Even the family does so: "Father James, I'm Dick"—so he doesn't have to try to guess. Everyone coming in reminds him of where he is, what the day and date are, what the time is and the next meal ("You'll soon have lunch") and so on. A day or so of this and the confusion and disorientation lift and the man is again just a normal elderly patient convalescing from hip surgery and can now be treated as such.

It's a technique any family can use—and should demand that the hospital and its staff follow, too, to protect the older patient at such a time of stress. RO can prevent an elderly person from becoming disoriented and confused and, as we have seen, can also be effective for those who are already disoriented.

The basis of RO, Dr. Folsom explains, is "to behave in relationship to the patient as though you expect him to participate in his own recovery and as though you have every expectation that he will be able to get his life back in shape again. . . . I've seen patients who didn't know their own name or what year or even what century it was, but after twenty-four-hour-a-day reality orientation, keeping a calm environment, reminding them who they were and where they were and why and literally what their name was at every contact—and even creating contacts to get patients oriented to their environments—I've seen these people change, *know* who they were, where they were, where the other significant people in their lives were and whether these people existed any more. It's a humanization process, a process of giving meaning back to the lives of these people."

The older patient for whom RO is used has often totally withdrawn into himself, cut personal relationships, and lost all awareness and interest. Dr. Folsom believes that even those parts of the brain that are still able to function have ground to a halt and what RO attempts to do is reactivate those unused neuronal pathways and help the patient develop new ways of functioning to compensate for the impairments that have occurred. To accomplish this, RO stimulates the person around the clock with reality ("today is Monday, it is now three o'clock, the next meal is dinner"). Formal thirty-minute classes raise the level of his functioning by increasingly difficult kinds of activities. The members of the group (usually few in number) are drilled in their names and those of the others, the day and the date. When such simple material has been absorbed, more difficult material is attacked—reading, writing, puzzles, discussions of the time of year or holidays, TV programs, or whatever is likely to help supply reality.

In an institution or a home, the entire staff and family participate in this total everyday push. For instance, as in the hospital example given earlier, the nurse or aide or porter will enter the room and announce his or her name and why he or she is there and use the patient's name: "Mr. Jones, I'm Miss Smith and I'm here to . . . It's ten o'clock now and you will eat lunch at twelve-thirty." The family may do it with, "Well, Jim, here I am, your wife, Mary, again. . . ." A big calendar with the days and dates marked off daily and a large clock are invariably kept visible, and a so-called "reality board" with changeable letters in large block characters will usually have the following posted on it for the purposes of drilling the patients (it may even be taken to the bedside):

THE NAME OF THIS PLACE IS ....[HOME]
TODAY IS ....
THE DATE IS ....
THE YEAR IS ....
THE TIME IS ....
THE NEXT MEAL IS ....
TOMORROW IS ....
THE COMING HOLIDAY IS ....

Blackboards are also frequently used for this purpose. Most agree that the best approach to the patient is a nonchallenging one: "Good morning, Mr. Brown," and not "Who are you?" or "What is your name?"; but some places do advocate direct questions, with the answers corrected and the person drilled in the correct answers. All of these methods may be varied according to the particular institution or home, for those utilizing RO tend to modify or add to it as seems best in the circumstances.

That RO works has been proven. Kenneth Pommerenck, a social worker in community organization and now a member of Dr. Folsom's ICD team, was instrumental in introducing RO into hospitals, nursing homes, and other facilities in New York State in 1968. The lady in her nineties, at the beginning of this chapter, was part of an experimental project Mr. Pommerenck introduced into a veterans home in which twenty-eight residents were provided with round-the-clock RO, while an equal number got the usual care provided by the home. Of those given RO, the number of those with severe or moderate disorientation was dramatically cut in half—but those who were treated as before remained essentially unchanged. The study lasted sixty days but the improvements seemed to continue afterward—and RO had been retained as the permanent practice of the home.

A two-year study has been carried out by investigators at the Maimonides Hospital and Home for the Aged in Montreal, Canada. A group of patients with severe chronic OBS and a mean age of eighty-two was divided into two groups similar in age, sex, and degree of problem. Over the two-year period one group was given conventional care while the other received RO—and those with the RO showed an improvement that was both statistically significant and clinically apparent.

There is good news as well for those families who wish to keep their loved ones at home even when they suffer OBS. This desire is now being made more practical thanks to the new community health centers that are springing up everywhere across the United States. Since July 1977 these centers have been required to provide an identifiable geriatric service, though there are as yet no specific requirements for their composition. Let's take a look at what these centers have to offer.

Mrs. Miriam Aronson, a gerontologist and associate in

psychiatry at Albert Einstein Medical School, is the director of the geriatric unit at the Soundview-Throgs Neck Community Mental Health Center, located in the north Bronx, New York City. Her unit, which has won an award from the National Council of Community Health Centers, offers its own modifications of RO. Twice a week, Mrs. Aronson (soon to be Dr. Aronson) has her patients discuss the day of the week, the month of the year, the holidays, what's going on in general, what's on TV, what the patients did that day—all in an effort to keep them oriented: "The whole purpose is to keep these people in the community." She also conducts simple crafts activities.

The RO props here include a large clock and a blackboard, plus her own touch—decorations of the season—the kind of individual difference that each program shows and that each family can use at home. Mrs. Aronson emphasizes again that to succeed, RO must be a twenty-four-hour-a-day affair with families or neighbors or friends pitching in to help at the very least "maintain the disoriented at a level of disorientation which may be less than if you ignored them."

Community mental health centers like Mrs. Aronson's provide the trained workers who can set the RO pattern and then work with the family as they follow the routine at home. They can provide the expertise and understanding needed to help the OBS victim perform a simple task—cooking potatoes, for instance. Typically, the task will be broken up into three stages: first, the family provides the potatoes and a peeler; once successfully peeled, a knife is supplied with instructions to cut the potatoes; once cut, the patient can proceed to the third stage of actual cooking. By proceeding step by step, the OBS victim can comprehend and cope with each separate job, and eventually may be able to put them all together into one unit.

The question that most often concerns families, though, is whether it is best to keep the OBS patient at home.

HOME OR INSTITUTION FOR THE OBS SUFFERER?

Sir Ferguson Anderson, one of Scotland's most eminent geriatricians, asserts, "It is likely that these patients deteriorate more rapidly in hospital." Dr. Libow agrees: "Institutionalization definitely has a negative effect, no one would argue with that. It's better to be in the community than in an institution and if I had my total choice there would be no institutions—*if* the society were willing to keep a human approach to those members with OBS who are remaining in the community." Most other experts would concur.

With the help of RO, it may be possible for the sufferer with OBS to be sufficiently reoriented to remain in the community. This is where the community mental health center's geriatric unit may be so vital, for its professional staff can support and advise those keeping patients at home; so well, in fact, that the care can be maintained without undue inconvenience for these supportive relations and friends.

Finally, there is Mrs. Aronson's note: "There is a very small minority for whom the nursing home or even the state hospital is quite appropriate. But the whole push today is to provide a whole range of options and the last one is institutionalization—the wave of the future is that the people who go to an institution will do so by *choice* and not by default."

THE OTHER VIEW

There are those who see the picture somewhat differently and who are more cautious about the uses of RO. Dr. Libow views chronic OBS as a "disease of unknown origin, and some day when we discover its cause we'll learn that there is a treatment that can prevent or reverse it." As for now, "There is at present no dramatic treatment but there are things that can be done to diminish its severity."

The dream of a cure, of a "magic bullet" or "miracle drug" for the dementias is an old one, and currently there are a few drugs that some experts feel may offer some help. There are many questions about their use, however, and none has been shown to be dramatically effective or of absolute proven value.

RO, however, *can* produce material changes in some sufferers even if it may not be regarded as a total cure, and so, until that wonderful day when some new drug makes it possible to cure senile dementia with a simple shot or pill, we might well listen to Dr. Folsom. He says of OBS and "senility": "I'd be willing to take anybody's cases, or have a treatment team like the one that existed when I was in Tuscaloosa put these people into an RO setting, and I believe we would have a remarkable turnaround in the vast majority of these cases." The large number of facilities throughout the country using his techniques every day would seem to agree with him.

So even if it is not the ultimate cure, there is at least some hope, something that can be done, for what was once called irreversible "senility." With expert professional help, families themselves can use RO at home and hope to bring the OBS of at least some sufferers under enough control so that they can *remain* at home.

There is still much to be done, however. In the words of one of the leading researchers in this field, Dr. Sinex: "It's not an impossible problem, not even a particularly complicated problem, but it's got to be brought out of the closet like cancer and you've got to talk about it. It's solvable—given enough money!" If the public demands an answer and supports the work still needed, some day, perhaps, "senility"—in *all* its manifestations—will be a thing of the past.

CHAPTER 10

Sources of Help and Information: Where To Find The Things That Matter

THE OLDER person is a member of virtually the most deprived minority in our country today. Neither his younger fellow citizens nor his doctor nor his political representatives are really interested in him, apart from the exceptional few; he is discriminated against both through ignorance and prejudice; he is even denied equality under the law in many ways—so it is essential that he know how to protect himself and where to find the help he needs.

This book has already attempted to help in certain areas, but each day brings new developments of importance to the over-sixty-five. Listed below are a group of organizations of vital importance to the older American: associations, institutes, and centers that will make it possible for him finally to swing some weight, to secure his rights, to keep abreast of new knowledge about legal, scientific, medical and social matters of interest to him. Some of the organizations are private and some governmental, but all are important. Also listed are some sources for postretirement jobs.

In parentheses will be found the addresses and even some specific persons or contacts to write to.

AMERICAN ASSOCIATION OF RETIRED PERSONS (AARP) (Mr. Lloyd Wright, Public Relations, AARP, 1909 K Street, N.W., Washington, D.C. 20049): This is surely the key organization for virtually every area of importance to the American fifty-five years of age and older. Three dollars a year pays for a joint membership for husband and wife, and with it this nonprofit, nonpartisan organization provides a vast range of services, from information of all kinds for the older American to lobbying (legislators are finally being made aware of the fact that some twenty-three million Americans are being short-changed politically, economically, and socially) to public information programs for those who still cling to the myths of senility and ageism. AARP representatives are recognized and respected when they go up to the Hill to speak before Congressional committees as the voice of the elderly, and its more-than-twenty-year-old fight against ageism has finally borne fruit with the recent bill raising the mandatory retirement age to seventy, and the complete prohibition of this practice in Florida and California.

Particularly noteworthy is its bimonthly magazine,

Modern Maturity, edited by an outstanding professional editor, Hubert C. Pryor, a former editor of *Look* and *Science Digest*. *Modern Maturity* is the only major national magazine concerning itself with the reality of the over-fifty-five person—what he and she are actually doing, what they need to know, what is happening for their benefit.

This magazine is only one of the publications offered by AARP, however. It also has a monthly newsletter of tabloid size to keep its members abreast of day-to-day happenings, and a flock of guidebooks on virtually everything that concerns the over-fifty-five American, from health to crime protection to food to taxes to legal problems. With nearly 30,000 local chapters, AARP also provides socialization to offset the loneliness of aging, health and automobile insurance, a Widowed Persons Service, an Institute of Lifetime Learning, buying services, and many other aids.

NATIONAL RETIRED TEACHERS ASSOCIATION (NRTA) (same address as AARP): In 1947, Dr. Ethel Percy Andrus, a retired Los Angeles High School principal and a social activist, founded this organization to fight for teachers' benefits and protection; it was from this background that she proceeded to found AARP and *Modern Maturity* in 1958. NRTA shares in virtually all the programs of AARP and the stationery carries both names, but NRTA has its own bi-monthly *NRTA Journal* for the specialized interest of teachers, with the same editor as *Modern Maturity*. There is also an NRTA monthly newsletter with material of special interest to teachers of fifty-five and older. Joining either organization provides virtually identical benefits.

NATIONAL INSTITUTE ON AGING (NIA) (Ms. Jane E. Shure, Public Information Officer, NIA, Bethesda, Md. 20014): One of the eleven Institutes of the National Institutes of Health, NIA's area of interest covers all aspects of aging. Thanks to the inspiration of its director, Dr. Robert N. Butler, NIA seeks to improve the quality of life for older Americans through biomedical, social, and behavioral research. Pamphlets and reports are increasingly available and a letter to NIA will bring a supply of authoritative information on virtually anything related to the elderly. It is particularly useful for current medical and medically related problems.

ICD REHABILITATION AND RESEARCH CENTER (ICD Registrar, 340 East 24th Street, New York, N.Y. 10010): ICD was the first rehabilitation center in the United States (it was founded in 1917) and its new director, Dr. James C. Folsom, has made this the Northeast U.S. Center for education and training in Reality Orientation (RO) and Attitude Therapy. Since its inception as a center for the vocational training of disabled World War I "doughboys," ICD has led in rehabilitation research and services and is now exploring many new services for the elderly. A letter will bring information on any of these.

DUKE UNIVERSITY CENTER FOR THE STUDY OF AGING AND HUMAN DEVELOPMENT (Duke University Medical Center, Box 3003, Durham, N.C. 27710): This was the first regional center in the country designated by the U.S. Public Health Service for the study of aging and it is now in its third decade of research. It serves older people in many ways through its research and clinic services (the Older Americans Resources and Services Division), the

Duke Institute for Learning in Retirement, and a wide variety of publications. A letter will bring information on this leading gerontological center.

GERONTOLOGY RESEARCH CENTER (GRC) (Daniel S. Rogers, Information Officer, GRC, Baltimore City Hospitals, Baltimore, Md. 21224): Established in 1940, this is the research facility of NIA. Since 1959 it has been carefully observing 650 active men (twenty to ninety-six years of age) to learn more about aging, how we can reduce disabilities and improve the everyday life of Americans. A source of much basic information.

ETHEL PERCY ANDRUS GERONTOLOGY CENTER (University of Southern California in Los Angeles, Los Angeles, Calif. 90007): Built by the donation of more than two million dollars from AARP and NRTA members, this major center of research and study into aging, with its Leonard Davis School of Gerontology (and many of its own students over sixty-five), provides a vast focus of knowledge and information. It even conducts clinical research on subjects such as memory training for older people, and is an excellent source of information, training, and learning for older people.

AMERICAN AGING ASSOCIATION (AGE) (c/o Dr. Denham Harman, 42nd and Dewey Avenue, Omaha, Neb. 68105): A national organization of laymen and scientists whose major goal is to increase the length of healthy, productive life through biomedical research. Its meetings bring together many of the leading scientists and researchers in gerontology.

NATIONAL INSTITUTE OF MENTAL HEALTH (NIMH) (Public Inquiries Branch, NIMH, Parklawn Bldg., 5600 Fishers Lane, Rockville, Md. 20857): NIMH covers the mental health of all Americans, and in such areas as depression and suicide may offer more material than NIA. A letter will bring material.

NATIONAL CLEARINGHOUSE FOR ALCOHOL INFORMATION (P.O. Box 2345, Rockville, Md. 20852): This is the source for information on alcohol problems. A letter will bring results.

NATIONAL INTERFAITH COALITION ON AGING (NICA) (Mr. Thomas C. Cook, NICA, 298 S. Hull St., Athens, Ga. 30605): NICA strives to develop the widest possible help for older Americans through the resources and help of our religions as well as such nonreligious groups as AARP-NRTA and various educational centers. NICA national conferences are highly regarded by many gerontologists. A letter will bring any information desired.

AMERICAN CANCER SOCIETY: The local chapters have considerable information on a wide range of self-help material and services, such as their "Reach to Recovery" program for those who have recovered from such surgery as mastectomies, laryngectomies, and the like.

THE NATIONAL COUNCIL ON THE AGING (1828 L Street, N.W., Washington, D.C. 20036): This organization offers a wide variety of aids, programs, and publications of help to older Americans. A letter will bring information.

GRAY PANTHERS (3700 Chestnut Street, Philadelphia, Pennsylvania, 10904). An immensely valuable activist network of older people. They lobby Washington, put out a newspaper called *Network*, hold consciousness-raising sessions, and in general fight for the rights and needs of the elderly. You may be able to find (or found) local chapters in your area. Write for information.

INTERNATIONAL SENIOR CITIZENS ASSOCIATION (11753 Wilshire Blvd., Los Angeles, Calif. 90025): For those interested in what their peers are doing elsewhere in the world; a letter will bring information.

STATE AND LOCAL OFFICES FOR THE AGING Most states and many localities have these under a variety of titles. Such agencies often provide a great deal of valuable information. The telephone book or the local library will furnish names and addresses.

SPECIAL WORK PROGRAMS FOR THE RETIRED

There are a variety of government-sponsored programs that provide opportunities for older Americans to find productive, useful roles in our society. ACTION is the name of the federal voluntary service agency that opens the way for older Americans to serve full or part time, on a volunteer or paid basis. Some positions provide expenses, others none, and there may be benefits such as accident insurance, health examinations, and the like.

ACTION: For information, write ACTION, Office of Public Affairs, 806 Connecticut Ave., N.W., Washington,

D.C. 20525—or call their toll-free number, 800-424-8580. The programs are:

RETIRED SENIOR VOLUNTEER PROGRAM (RSVP): Retired persons sixty years and older can utilize their talents and experience here. They may serve without compensation, but with expenses paid, in a variety of organizations, agencies and institutions such as courts, schools, libraries, hospitals, and community service centers. The tasks are very varied.

FOSTER GRANDPARENTS PROGRAM: A program designed for those with low incomes, but the standards for "low income" vary widely. Participants receive financial assistance and a variety of side benefits for providing companionship and guidance to mentally, physically, or emotionally handicapped children.

SENIOR COMPANION PROGRAM: Also for low-income people. Participants receive a stipend for helping adults and elderly people with shopping, assistance in securing medical and other social services, and other such jobs.

PEACE CORPS and VISTA: Both programs are open to older people with special skills or knowledge interested in serving either in the developing countries or with our own deprived groups in the United States. There is a monthly stipend and other benefits.

We will end our book with a quotation from the writing of the late Dr. Ethel Percy Andrus: "Old age is not a defeat but a victory, not a punishment but a privilege." When all Americans recognize this, we will have ended ageism and laid to rest the myths of senility and of old age.

Bibliography and Selected Readings

Anderson, Sir F. *Practical Management of the Elderly*. 3d ed. Oxford, England: Blackwell Scientific Publications, 1976.

Atkinson, R.C. and R.M. Shiffrin. "The Control of Short-Term Memory." *Scientific American*, August, 1971.

Berezin, M.A. and S.H. Cath. *Geriatric Psychiatry*. New York: International Universities Press, 1965.

Botwinick, J. *Aging and Behavior*. New York: Springer Publishing, 1973.

Bourne, G.H. "The Aging Process." *The Yerkes Newsletter*,February, 1975.

Brown, B.S. "Interview," *MH*, Summer, 1975.

Busse, E.W. "Hypochondriasis in the Elderly." *J. Am. Geriatr. Soc.*, April, 1976.

——— and E. Pfeiffer. *Behavior and Adaptation in Late Life*. Boston: Little, Brown, 1977.

Butler, R.N. *Why Survive*. New York: Harper & Row, 1975.

——— and M.I. Lewis. *Aging and Mental Health*. 2d ed. St. Louis: C.V. Mosby, 1977.

———. *Sex After Sixty*. New York: Harper & Row, 1976.

Byrd, G.J. "Acute Organic Brain Syndrome Associated with Gentamicin Therapy." *J.A.M.A.*, July 4, 1977.

Cohen, S. "Geriatric Drug Abuse." Paper presented at Vista Hill Foundation Seminar, February, 1975.

Committee on Human Sexuality, A.M.A. *Human Sexuality.* Chicago: A.M.A., 1972.

Davis, J.M. "Which Patients Need ECT?" *Medical World News*, October 27, 1975.

Ferlemann, M. "The Golden Years." *Menninger Perspective*, June/July, 1972.

Folsom, J.C. and G.S. Folsom. "The Real World." *MH*, Summer, 1974.

______ and L.R. Taulbee. "Reality Orientation for Geriatric Patients." *Hospital & Community Psychiatry*, May, 1966.

Frederick, C.J. and L. Lague. *Dealing with the Crisis of Suicide.* Public Affairs Pamphlet No. 406A, 1972.

Hamlin, R.M. "Restrictions on the Competent Aged." Paper presented at American Psychological Association Annual Convention, August 26, 1977.

Henig, R.M. "Tomorrow's Challenge: Health Care for the Elderly." *The New Physician*, October, 1977.

Hoffman, A.M. *The Daily Needs and Interests of Older People.* Springfield, Ill.: Charles C Thomas, 1976.

Howells, J.G. *Modern Perspectives in the Psychiatry of Old Age.* New York: Brunner/Mazel, 1975.

Kahn, R.L., et al. "Memory Complaint and Impairment in the Aged." *Arch. Gen. Psychiatry,* December, 1975.

Knowles, John. *Doing Better and Feeling Worse: Health in the United States.* W.W. Norton, 1977.

Leaf, A. "Getting Old." *Scientific American,* September, 1973.

Leshner, M. and A. Goldman. "Sexual Barriers in the Aged." Paper presented at American Psychological Association Annual Convention, September, 1974.

Libow, L.S. "Pseudo-Senility." *J. Am. Geriatr. Soc.*, March, 1973.

Masters, M.W. and V.E. Johnson. "Sex after Sixty." *Medical World News*, (*Geriatrics* 1971 issue).

Mathews, M.V. et al. "Exploring the Speed of Mental Processes." *Bell Laboratories Record*, March, 1975.

McCary, J.L. *Sexual Myths and Fallacies.* New York: Van Nostrand Reinhold, 1971.

Menninger, K.A. "Old Age without Depression." *Medical World News*, (*Geriatrics* 1971 issue).

National Institute of Mental Health: *It's Good To Know About Mental Health.* 1973.

Ostfeld, A.M. and D.C. Gibson. *Epidemiology of Aging.* U.S. Department of Health, Education, and Welfare. HEW Publication (NIH) 75-711.

Palmore, E. *Normal Aging.* Durham, N.C.: Duke University Press, 1970.

———. *Normal Aging II.* Durham, N.C.: Duke University Press, 1974.

Parry, H.J. et al. "National Patterns of Psychotherapeutic Drug Use." *Arch. Gen. Psychiatry*, June 1973.

Patten, B.M. "Improve Your Memory." AMA *Update*, Christmas, 1972.

Peak, D.T. "Mental Health." Paper presented at the A.M.A. Quality of Life Congress—the Later Years, 1974.

Penfield, W. *The Mystery of the Mind.* Princeton, N.J.: Princeton University Press, 1975.

Pfeiffer, E. *Successful Aging: A Conference Report.* Durham, N.C.: Duke University Center for the Study of Aging, 1974.

———. "Successful Aging." Paper presented at the A.M.A. Quality of Life Congress—the Later Years, 1974.

Rubin, I. *Sexual Life After Sixty.* New York: Basic Books, 1965.

Shank, R.E. "Nutrition and Aging." From *Epidemiology of Aging.* U.S. Department of Health, Education, and Welfare. HEW Publication (NIH) 75-711.

Shneidman, E.S. *Suicidology: Contemporary Developments.* New York: Grune & Stratton, 1976.

Squire, L.R. "Memory Functions Six to Nine Months after Electroconvulsive Therapy." *Arch. Gen. Psychiatry,* December, 1975.

Steinberg, F.U. *Cowdry's The Care of the Geriatric Patient.* 5th ed. St. Louis: C.V. Mosby, 1976.

Terry, R.D. "Dementia: A Brief and Selective Review." *Arch. Neurol.*, January, 1976.

Wetzel, R.D. "Hopelessness, Depression, and Suicide Intent." *Arch. Gen. Psychiatry*, September, 1976.

Index